Current Practices in Ophthalmology

Series Editor

Parul Ichhpujani
Department of Ophthalmology
Government Medical College and Hospital
Chandigarh, India

This series of highly organized and uniform handbooks aims to cover the latest clinically relevant developments in ophthalmology. In the wake of rapidly evolving innovations in the field of basic research, pharmacology, surgical techniques and imaging devices for the management of ophthalmic disorders, it is extremely important to invest in books that help you stay updated. These handbooks are designed to bridge the gap between journals and standard texts providing reviews on advances that are now part of mainstream clinical practice. Meant for residents, fellows-in-training, generalist ophthalmologists and specialists alike, each volume under this series covers current perspectives on relevant topics and meets the CME requirements as a go-to reference guide. Supervised and reviewed by a subject expert, chapters in each volume provide leading-edge information most relevant and useful for clinical ophthalmologists. This series is also useful for residents and fellows training in various subspecialties of ophthalmology, who can read these books while at work or during emergency duties. Additionally, these handbooks can aid in preparing for clinical case discussions at various forums and examinations.

More information about this series at http://www.springer.com/series/15743

Parul Ichhpujani • Manpreet Singh
Editors

Ophthalmic Instruments and Surgical Tools

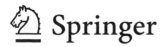 Springer

Editors
Parul Ichhpujani
Department of Ophthalmology
Government Medical College and Hospital
Chandigarh
India

Manpreet Singh
Department of Ophthalmology
Post Graduate Institute of Medical
Education and Research
Chandigarh
India

ISSN 2523-3807   ISSN 2523-3815   (electronic)
Current Practices in Ophthalmology
ISBN 978-981-13-7675-7   ISBN 978-981-13-7673-3   (eBook)
https://doi.org/10.1007/978-981-13-7673-3

© Springer Nature Singapore Pte Ltd. 2019
This work is subject to copyright. All rights are reserved by the Publisher, whether the whole or part of the material is concerned, specifically the rights of translation, reprinting, reuse of illustrations, recitation, broadcasting, reproduction on microfilms or in any other physical way, and transmission or information storage and retrieval, electronic adaptation, computer software, or by similar or dissimilar methodology now known or hereafter developed.
The use of general descriptive names, registered names, trademarks, service marks, etc. in this publication does not imply, even in the absence of a specific statement, that such names are exempt from the relevant protective laws and regulations and therefore free for general use.
The publisher, the authors, and the editors are safe to assume that the advice and information in this book are believed to be true and accurate at the date of publication. Neither the publisher nor the authors or the editors give a warranty, expressed or implied, with respect to the material contained herein or for any errors or omissions that may have been made. The publisher remains neutral with regard to jurisdictional claims in published maps and institutional affiliations.

This Springer imprint is published by the registered company Springer Nature Singapore Pte Ltd.
The registered company address is: 152 Beach Road, #21-01/04 Gateway East, Singapore 189721, Singapore

Foreword

It is with great pleasure that I write this foreword to the book, *Ophthalmic Instruments and Surgical Tools*, edited by Drs Parul Ichhpujani and Manpreet Singh, who I have known for several years to be highly motivated and enthusiastic young ophthalmic surgeons and teachers. I congratulate them for taking this initiative for filling a long felt gap on the availabilty of current information on ophthalmic surgical instruments, their uses, sterilization, and their upkeep. In the ever-changing world of the surgical techniques in ophthalmology, a description of surgical instruments has remained neglected in the past so many decades. The young ophthalmic surgeons, trainees, and students are often at a loss to find information on the instruments and equipment before they start using these. The editors have succeeded in filling this gap admirably well. The editors have complied a roster of young ophthalmic faculty members to contribute chapters on the surgical instruments and equipment used in a variety of surgical procedures in the anterior segment, vitreoretinal surgery, and the oculoplastic and orbital surgery.

A dedicated text on the planned compilation, lucid description, pertinent uses, and intraoperative handling of the surgical instruments used in specialty ophthalmic surgeries is rare. Moreover, the photographs of instruments from various aspects provide a clearer image in the minds of readership for better understandings. This book will be a remarkable addition to the literature and of interest not only to the ophthalmologists under training but also to the nursing staff and undergraduate students.

The make, material, description, and sterilization of a surgical instrument are often overlooked and ignored entity. The surgical instruments are mostly "looked-at" and read by the students before exams with great difficulties in collecting the information and remembering afresh as an entirely new aspect. This book will go a long way in helping the readership in educating nursing staff, students, residents, fellows, and clinicians in practice.

Chandigarh, India   Amod Gupta

Acknowledgements

Mrs. Surjit Kaur (ANS), Mrs. Seema Rani, Mr. Sandeep Kumar, Mrs. Mary Daisy, Mrs. Chin L Hatlang, and Mr. Rajesh—Operation theatre nursing officers, Advanced Eye Centre, PGIMER, Chandigarh—for providing clean and organized instruments/ equipment.

Dr. Kuldeep Raizada and Mrs. Deepa Raizada—Akriti Oculoplasty Logistics, Hyderabad, Telangana, India—for providing pictures of rare surgical instruments.

Contents

About the Editors

Parul Ichhpujani is currently an Associate Professor in the Department of Ophthalmology at Government Medical College and Hospital, Chandigarh, India, where she is chiefly responsible for glaucoma and neuro-ophthalmology services. She completed her glaucoma training at the Advanced Eye Centre of Postgraduate Institute of Medical Education and Research (PGIMER), Chandigarh, India, and in a subsequent Clinical Research fellowship, under Dr. George L Spaeth, at Wills Eye Institute, Philadelphia, USA. She currently serves on the Education Committee of the World Glaucoma Association and is the Associate Managing Editor of the *Journal of Current Glaucoma Practice*, the official journal of the International Society of Glaucoma Surgery. She was ranked among the Powerlist 2015 for the "Best 40 ophthalmologists under 40."An avid researcher, Dr. Ichhpujani has coauthored three books: *Pearls in Glaucoma Therapy*, *Living with Glaucoma*, and *Smart Resources in Ophthalmology*; and has edited another five: *Expert Techniques in Ophthalmology*, *Glaucoma: Basic and Clinical Perspectives*, *Manual of Glaucoma*, *Clinical Cases in Glaucoma: An Evidence Based Approach*, and *Glaucoma: Intraocular Pressure and Aqueous Dynamics*. She has contributed several research articles and book chapters in national and international books and serves as a reviewer for many ophthalmology journals.

Manpreet Singh is currently an Assistant Professor in the Department of Ophthalmology at the Postgraduate Institute of Medical Education and Research (PGIMER), Chandigarh, India, where he is responsible for ophthalmic plastic surgery services. After completing his senior residency at PGIMER, he pursued a fellowship in Oculofacial Aesthetics at Sri Sankaradeva Nethralaya, Guwahati, India, with Dr. Kasturi Bhattacharjee. Later, he worked as a fellow with Dr. Mohd. Javed Ali at LV Prasad Eye Institute, Hyderabad, India, and learned various endoscopic endonasal lacrimal procedures. Dr. Singh serves as a reviewer for various national and international journals and has published over 35 papers and one book chapter.

Contributors

Monika Balyan Cataract and Refractive Services, Department of Ophthalmology, Advanced Eye Centre, Post Graduate Institute of Medical Education and Research (PGIMER), Chandigarh, India

Mohit Dogra Vitreo-Retina Services, Department of Ophthalmology, Advanced Eye Centre, Post Graduate Institute of Medical Education and Research (PGIMER), Chandigarh, India

Natasha Gautam Glaucoma Services, Department of Ophthalmology, Advanced Eye Centre, Post Graduate Institute of Medical Education and Research (PGIMER), Chandigarh, India

Priya Goyal Glaucoma Services, Department of Ophthalmology, Government Medical College and Hospital, Chandigarh, India

Aditi Mehta Grewal Cataract and Refractive Services, Department of Ophthalmology, Advanced Eye Centre, Post Graduate Institute of Medical Education and Research (PGIMER), Chandigarh, India

Sartaj Singh Grewal Grewal Eye Institute, Chandigarh, India

Amit Gupta Cataract and Refractive Services, Department of Ophthalmology, Advanced Eye Centre, Post Graduate Institute of Medical Education and Research (PGIMER), Chandigarh, India

Varshitha Hemanth Clinical Fellow in Ophthalmic Plastic Surgery, Ocular Oncology and Socket Sciences, L V Prasad Eye Institute (LVPEI), Hyderabad, India

Parul Ichhpujani Glaucoma Services, Department of Ophthalmology, Government Medical College and Hospital, Chandigarh, India

Arun K. Jain Cataract and Refractive Services, Department of Ophthalmology, Advanced Eye Centre, Post Graduate Institute of Medical Education and Research (PGIMER), Chandigarh, India

Sahil Jain Department of Ophthalmology, Advanced Eye Centre, Post Graduate Institute of Medical Education and Research (PGIMER), Chandigarh, India

Saurabh Kamal Ophthalmic Plastic Surgeon, Eyehub, Faridabad, Haryana, India

Deeksha Katoch Department of Ophthalmology, Advanced Eye Centre, Post Graduate Institute of Medical Education and Research (PGIMER), Chandigarh, India

Manpreet Kaur Glaucoma Services, Department of Ophthalmology, Advanced Eye Centre, Post Graduate Institute of Medical Education and Research (PGIMER), Chandigarh, India

Chintan Malhotra Cataract and Refractive Services, Department of Ophthalmology, Advanced Eye Centre, Post Graduate Institute of Medical Education and Research (PGIMER), Chandigarh, India

Jagjit Malhotra Advanced Eye Centre, Post Graduate Institute of Medical Education and Research (PGIMER), Chandigarh, India

Natasha Gautam Seth Glaucoma Services, Department of Ophthalmology, Advanced Eye Centre, Post Graduate Institute of Medical Education and Research (PGIMER), Chandigarh, India

Manpreet Singh Oculoplastics Services, Department of Ophthalmology, Advanced Eye Centre, Post Graduate Institute of Medical Education and Research (PGIMER), Chandigarh, India

Prerana Tahiliani Oculoplastics and Ocular Oncology, Mumbai Eye Plastic Surgery, Mumbai, India

Anchal Thakur Cataract and Refractive Services, Department of Ophthalmology, Advanced Eye Centre, Post Graduate Institute of Medical Education and Research (PGIMER), Chandigarh, India

Sahil Thakur Department of Ocular Epidemiology, Singapore Eye Research Institute, Singapore

Sonam Yangzes Cataract and Refractive Services, Department of Ophthalmology, Advanced Eye Centre, Post Graduate Institute of Medical Education and Research (PGIMER), Chandigarh, India

Instrument Sterilization and Care

1

Manpreet Singh and Jagjit Malhotra

The operation theatre equipment, machines, trolleys, and surgical instruments demand extra care as compared to other areas. The cleaning, disinfection, and sterilization of these items depend upon their role in the operation or surgery. Of these, the most frequently circulated and used items are the surgical instruments. Hence, proper cleaning, debridement, packing, and sterilization are of utmost importance before the use, repeat use, or storage of the instruments. Earle Spaulding (1968) from Philadelphia classified medical instruments, depending upon their use and risk of spreading infection. The instruments were grouped as critical, semi-critical, and noncritical devices (Table 1.1).

Table 1.1 Spaulding classification of instruments

Classification		Products	Cleaning process	Cleaning product
Critical	Enters inside sterile body cavities, bloodstream, or sterile tissue	Surgical instruments, implants, scalpel blades, needles, cannula, phacoemulsification handpieces	Sterilization	Sterilizing agent or process
Semi-critical	Comes in contact with non-sterile mucous membranes or non-intact skin	Endoscopes, the tip of applanation or indentation tonometer, the probe of contact/immersion biometry, Schirmer's strips, fluorescein strips, etc.	Sterilization or high-level disinfection	Sterilizing agent or process/disinfectant
Noncritical	Comes in contact with intact skin	Rulers, exophthalmometers, ultrasonography probes, blood-pressure cuffs	Low-level disinfection	Soap and water

M. Singh (✉)
Oculoplastics Services, Department of Ophthalmology, Advanced Eye Centre,
Post Graduate Institute of Medical Education and Research (PGIMER), Chandigarh, India

J. Malhotra
Deputy Nursing Superintendent, Advanced Eye Centre,
Post Graduate Institute of Medical Education and Research (PGIMER), Chandigarh, India

© Springer Nature Singapore Pte Ltd. 2019
P. Ichhpujani, M. Singh (eds.), *Ophthalmic Instruments and Surgical Tools*,
Current Practices in Ophthalmology,
https://doi.org/10.1007/978-981-13-7673-3_1

The conventional ophthalmic instruments are fine and mostly blood-free and have delicate ends which require careful handling during the complete sterilization cycle as compared to other surgical specialties. On the contrary, the instruments used in ophthalmic plastic surgery invariably get bloodstained. Blood contains hemoglobin and iron (Fe) which get lodged into micro-abrasions or cracks of the instrument coatings and invoke rusting. Careful soap and water cleaning removes most of the dirt, blood clots, and microorganisms. Cold water is preferred over hot to prevent the heat coagulation of proteins over the instrument surface, making it difficult to remove. Without cleaning, the disinfection and sterilization remain ineffective.

1.1   Stepwise Processing of the Used Instruments

1.1.1   Cleaning

Cleaning is the physical removal of visible dirt, blood, pus, lint fibers, or threads from the instruments. For fine and delicate ophthalmic instruments, the mechanical cleaning is preferred over the manual one to minimize the instrument damage and for efficient performance. Moreover, it prevents the infectious hazard to the instrument handlers and saves time in a busy operation theatre. Always use distilled water (DW) for cleaning—the normal saline and balanced salt solutions damage the instrument coatings and joints by corrosion. Adequate ventilation with temperature and humidity control is desirable requirements for the cleaning area.

Ultrasonic cleaning (Fig. 1.1) is the most efficient and effective technique to clean instruments. The sound waves of frequency ≥100 KHz pass against the

Fig. 1.1 An ultrasonic cleaner with a bowl-tray to contain the instruments to be cleaned. The arrow highlights the 'inlet' for the water or solution

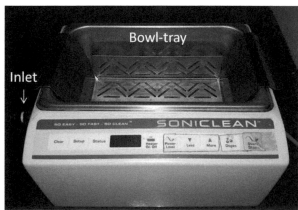

water-dipped instruments. Fine-tipped and delicate micro-instruments are advisable for ultrasonic cleaning. For ultrasonic cleaning, the neutral pH solution should be used which improves calibration and reduces the surface tension. The fluid should be changed daily or whenever required in 1 day.

(a) Turn on the machine for 8–10 min to get rid of any microbubbles from the solution before placing instruments (150 °F).
(b) Grossly clean the larger instruments before placing it inside the wire basket of ultrasonicator.
(c) Open box lock joints and ratchets for better effect.
(d) To prevent cross-plating or cross-metalling, do not overload or mix dissimilar metals.
(e) After completion of the cycle, remove the instruments, rinse them, and air-dry them.

After cleaning, rinsing of all instruments with DW should be done to remove the surface "biofilm." Rinsing of cannulas, vitreous cutters, tubings, and metallic suction tips with DW and air is a must. The lubrication is the next desirable step which prevents further sticking of proteins and improves "life" of the instrument. The lubrication of instruments with the lumen is not advisable.

1.1.2 Drying

Now, the instruments are dried with a lint-free cloth and regular hair dryer before the packing. At this time, the instruments should be inspected under magnification for tip and tooth alignment of forceps, cutting edges of scissors, approximation of needle holders, and suture tying forceps. Fine cleanliness, corrosion, cracks, pits, burrs, nicks, etc. are other observed details.

1.1.3 Packing or Wrapping

Rigid containers made up of metal, plastic, or aluminum are used to store most of the ophthalmic instruments. Transparent pouches and sterilization wraps (synthetic or organic fabric) are used wherever necessary.

The synthetic disposable wrapping material is preferred over woven textiles (Fig. 1.2). Fabric or textile drape cloth (Fig. 1.2) should have a minimum of 140 threads/inch^2, and minimum residual soap is desirable after washing of cloth. This prevents the soap deposits on instruments after autoclaving. Paper, polyolefin, peel-pack rolls, or pouches are used for packing the small boxes or individual instruments before sterilization.

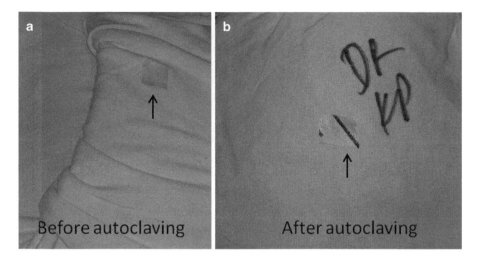

Fig. 1.2 (**a**) The arrow shows a blank sticker placed over the wrapped linen before autoclaving. (**b**) After autoclaving, the sticker shows a black stripe indicating the autoclaved lot

During packing or wrapping, the sterilization indicators (chemical or biological) are put inside the pouches for the assessment of sterilization adequacy. The storage plates should preferably have perforations for better steam penetration and effective drying during autoclaving. Always place heavier instruments at the bottom and lighter ones on top. The tip protectors should be used to safeguard the business-end tips of fine ophthalmic instruments. Approximately 1-inch space is kept around the boxes and plastic wrappers. The labeling of the package should clearly indicate the date of sterilization, lot number, contents, and initials of the sterilization processing person. The style of packaging must permit the presentation of the stored contents to the sterile area or trolley in a straightforward and aseptic manner.

1.1.4   Sterilization

The process of sterilization involves the complete destruction of all microorganisms and the spores. Disinfection means killing or destruction of microorganisms only. Various methods of sterilization include autoclaving, hot air oven, ethylene oxide (ETO) gas, plasma sterilization (hydrogen peroxide gas), and chemical agents like glutaraldehyde 2%. Out of these, autoclaving, ETO, and plasma are commonly used sterilization methods in ophthalmology. A simple test known as *Bowie-Dick test* is used to assess the penetration of steam till the middle of a test sack made up of cotton towels. An autoclave test tape indicator is placed in the center, and a test cycle is run—a uniform change (from beige to brown) of the tape indicates adequate penetration of steam. As also mentioned by the manufacturers, this is not the perfect test to guarantee sterilization. The salient features of the following methods have been summarized and compiled in Table 1.2.

Table 1.2 Techniques for sterilization

Technique	Merits	Demerits	Time and temperature	Ideal for
Autoclave (pressurized steam)	• Inexpensive • Highly effective • Rapid • Nontoxic	• Not suitable for oils, powder, ointment, etc. • Closed glass chambers • Rubber, plastic can melt	20–60 min 121–180 °C	• Operating metallic instruments • Surgical gowns, drapes, dressings
Hot air oven (dry heat)	• Non-corrosive • Inexpensive Nontoxic	• Less effective • Longer duration	60–80 min 340 °F	• Oils, powder, etc. • Metallic instruments • Open glass vials
Ethylene oxide (ETO)	• Heat-labile tubes • Plastic handle blades • Wires • Longer storage • Ready to use pack	• Toxic • Expensive • Caution for handlers (carcinogenic, explosive) • Long cycle time • Long aeration time	6–12 h	• Vitrectomy cutters • Phaco tubings • Optical-fiber light pipe • Silicone stents • Acrylic orbital implants • Conformers • Plastic eye shields • Cryoprobes
Plasma (hydrogen peroxide)	• Short cycle time • Ready to use • Plastic, heat-labile material • Wires • Longer storage	• Special packing needed • Expensive equipment	75–80 min	Same as of ETO
Chemical disinfectants	• Quick and ready method • Inexpensive	• Not for any intraocular instrument • Needs thorough wash for all items • Proper lumen rinsing before use • Toxic to mucosa and conjunctiva	3–4 h	• Nasal endoscope tips • Nasal packing forceps • Plastic, glass, airways, etc.

- *Autoclaves*: These (Fig. 1.3) use the compressed or pressurized steam as a sterilizing agent. It is an inexpensive, nontoxic, easy, expedient, and efficient method of sterilization. The packaged trays should be arranged for adequate steam surround and penetration. After switching on, the air inside autoclave is removed by

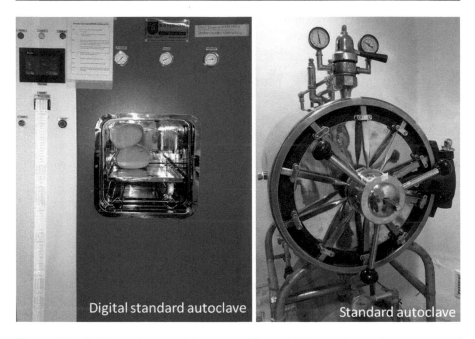

Fig. 1.3 The digital autoclave containing wrapped linen with the autoclave cycle parameters and timings recorded on a printed strip. The standard autoclave shows analogue gauges and meters with no record of previous cycles.

the vacuum pump and is replaced by the steam. The operating temperature and pressure are maintained and monitored externally by gauges. Total cycle time and other parameters should be according to the equipment manufacturer. Flash sterilizers are commonly used under emergency conditions, and items sterilized are recommended to be used immediately by most of the manufacturers.

- *Hot air oven*: This uses dry heat sterilization method. It is generally used to sterilize oil, ointment, powders, glass vials, and metal instruments. All items should be preferably dry. The items should be immediately used after cooling. Time taken for sterilization is generally more than an autoclave.
- *Ethylene oxide* (C_2H_4O): This is an alkalinizing agent toxic to the DNA of microbes. It is used mainly for the moisture and heat-sensitive devices. The concentration of gas, exposure time, temperature, and relative humidity are major functioning parameters. Proper documentation of each parameter is necessary for best efficiency and to avoid accidents. This method demands a lengthy aeration time (with filtered air) after every cycle for the removal of harmful residuals. This is done before opening the door of the machine. All sterilized items must be aerated properly before safe use as the residual contents can incite intraocular inflammation. Regular testing of the machine area is necessary to check for the gas exposure. The process is carried out at a temperature of 45–55 °C, relative humidity of 60%, and the pressure between 5 and 10 psi for 12–6 h, respectively.

- *Plasma sterilization*: Plasma sterilization (Fig. 1.4) uses hydrogen peroxide that is used in gas or vapor form. Plasma constitutes highly ionized gas composed of ionic particles (electrons, neutrons, etc.) produced by excitation of gas or vapors by radiofrequency or microwaves in a closed chamber under low-vacuum conditions. Plasma constitutes low-temperature sterilization in which polypropylene, polyolefin, and plastic have preferably used a packing or wrapping material. The cellulose content of paper and cloth absorbs the peroxide preventing its effective penetration.

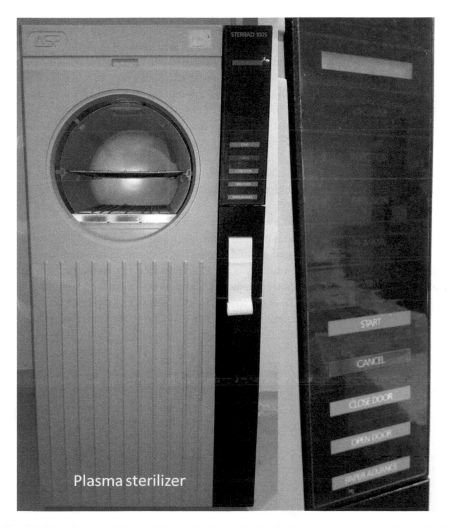

Fig. 1.4 The plasma sterilizer with 'open door' showing the shelves to keep the wrapped items. Each cycle is printed on the stripe for record maintenance. Various options and cycle stage indicators

- *Chemical sterilization*: *Glutaraldehyde 2%* is an effective sterilizing agent available in liquid form. Heat-labile equipment, endoscopes, and metal instruments are commonly placed into this solution for minimum 3 h. These instruments are thoroughly washed or rinsed before use. The solution should be replaced after 2 weeks.

   Isopropyl alcohol (70%)—It is a low-cost disinfectant for ophthalmic lenses, tips of applanation or indentation tonometers, and other OPD or OT metallic instruments. It should be wiped dry before use and must be used with caution as it is highly inflammable. *Other chemical agents—Sodium hypochlorite, chlorhexidine*, and *10% povidone-iodine*.

   Formalin in the form of tablets, liquid, and aerosol is used for sterilization of many operation theatre items. The transparent, shelved, airtight box containing heat-sensitive equipment (wires, leads, endoscopes, fiber-optic light pipes, etc.) is generally used. The standard concentration used is 7 g/m^3. The shelves should preferably be perforated for better circulation of vapors. The box can be kept at room temperature. The sterilizing time is 12 h and the box should not be opened during this time. Eye protection wear is helpful from this potentially carcinogenic chemical. In many institutions, its use has been discontinued due to its potential carcinogenicity.

1.2   Effective Sterilization Monitoring

It is always indirectly indicated by a few mechanical, chemical, and biological indicators (Fig. 1.5). The mechanical indicators are intra-process temperature, pressure, and time as depicted by the gauges and necessary documentation on charts. The chemical indicators are commonly used for ETO, autoclaving, and dry heat sterilization. These are commonly placed in the middle of items or packs where the steam might take longest to reach. These are available as adhesive tapes placed outside the packs making it easier to distinguish between an autoclaved and unsterile pack.

Fig. 1.5 A steam indicator (chemical) tape with the arrows showing the site of chemical stripe. The space in between two lines is used to label the date, time and signature of nursing officer

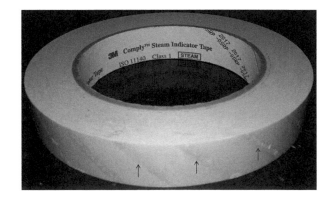

Table 1.3 Storage times for material sterilized by different methods of sterilization

Technique	Storage time/shelf life
Autoclave (pressurized steam)	72 h {only in a controlled environment having a temperature (20 °C–24 °C) and humidity (less than 60%)}
Hot air oven (dry heat)	Vary according to article/equipment
Ethylene oxide (ETO)	3 Months
Plasma (hydrogen peroxide)	6 Months
Chemical disinfectants	Vary according to disinfectant used

The biological indicators measure the effectiveness of sterilization at closest to the direct assessment. *Bacillus subtilis* spores are heat-resistant endospores, but when killed by the pressurized steam of autoclave, it is presumed that all other microorganisms must have been destroyed. After completion of the autoclave cycle, the strips containing endospores are incubated for 7 days. If no growth is demonstrated, the then autoclaved lot is considered to be sterile. This delay of the result is a considerable disadvantage making the chemical indicators as the most used ones.

Nonetheless, a comprehensive "operation theatre employees orientation program," proper documentation of the sterilization process, monitoring of sterilization, and written instructions have a vital role in running an efficient operation theatre.

Note Whenever there is doubt about the sterility of any instrument, equipment, or surgeon's wear, consider it unsterile and proceed accordingly.

1.3   Storage of Sterile Instruments and Linen

Good storage condition is utmost important. Instruments should be placed at least 2½ feet above the ground level. Shelves or storage racks should be carbolized and completely dry. Adequate temperature and humidity should be maintained. Keep a check on the expiry date of sterile material on a daily basis. Table 1.3 shows storage times for material sterilized by different methods of sterilization.

Suggested Reading

1. Burkhart NW, Crawford J. Critical steps in instrument cleaning: removing debris after sonication. J Am Dent Assoc. 1997;128(4):456–63.
2. Perakaki K, Mellor AC, Qualtrough AJ. Comparison of an ultrasonic cleaner and a washer disinfector in the cleaning of endodontic files. J Hosp Infect. 2007;67(4):355–9.
3. Seavey R. High-level disinfection, sterilization, and antisepsis: current issues in reprocessing medical and surgical instruments. Am J Infect Control. 2013;41(5 Suppl):S111–7.
4. Spruce L. Back to basics: instrument cleaning. AORN J. 2017;105(3):292–9.

Ophthalmic Sutures and Needles

2

Parul Ichhpujani and Priya Goyal

2.1 Definition

"Surgical suture" is a medical device that helps to approximate and hold body tissues after a surgery or an injury.

A surgical suture in ophthalmology is used for desired apposition of wound edges, hanging back of tissues (recti or levator), fixation of detached structures (canthal tendons, bones), and lifting of tissues (eyelid, facial skin). Moreover, suturing closes or reduces the dead space, hence decreasing the chances of hematoma collection and infection.

2.2 Ideal Suture Material

The ideal suture should have the following characteristics:

- Sterile
- Resistant to infection
- Have minimal tissue reaction; be nonallergenic and noncarcinogenic
- Favorable absorption profile
- Easy to handle
- Hold securely when knotted; must not fray or cut after knot is tied
- High tensile strength
- May be used for multiple types of tissues or surgical procedures
- Cheap

P. Ichhpujani (✉) · P. Goyal
Glaucoma Services, Department of Ophthalmology, Government Medical College and Hospital, Chandigarh, India

© Springer Nature Singapore Pte Ltd. 2019
P. Ichhpujani, M. Singh (eds.), *Ophthalmic Instruments and Surgical Tools*,
Current Practices in Ophthalmology,
https://doi.org/10.1007/978-981-13-7673-3_2

Despite technological advancements, even at present, there is no single material that befits all of the aforementioned characteristics.

2.3   Terminology Related to Sutures

Absorbable This refers to the loss of mass and/or volume of suture material over a period of time. It has no correlation with initial tensile strength of the suture material.

Nonabsorbable This refers to a material that is relatively immune to the biologic activities of the body tissues and stays unaltered at the surgical site unless removed.

Capillarity It is the extent to which absorbed fluid is transferred along the length of suture.

Fluid Absorption This refers to the ability of the suture material to take up fluid after immersion.

Breaking Strength This refers to the limit of tensile strength at which suture failure occurs.

Half-Life This refers to the time required for the tensile strength to reduce to its half of original value.

Knot-Pull Tensile Strength It is the breaking strength of knotted suture material.

Knot Strength Knot strength is the amount of force necessary to cause a knot to slip. The strength of a knotted suture usually decreases by 50% due to the stresses induced by bending and twisting. The coefficient of static friction and plasticity of a given material influences the knot strength.

Elasticity It is the measure of the ability of the suture material to regain its original form and length after deformation. High elasticity sutures are preferred for edematous tissues.

Memory Elasticity, plasticity, and diameter of a suture influence the inherent capability of a suture to return to or maintain its gross shape. A suture with a high degree of memory is stiff and may require an extra throw to prevent loosening of the knot.

Plasticity It is the measure of the ability to maintain its "new" form after stretching, without breaking.

Pliability This refers to the ease of handling of suture material and ability to adjust knot tension.

Tensile strength Tensile strength is the measure of the ability of a suture material to resist breakage and deformation.

Tensile strength depends upon the suture material and its diameter, condition of the suture (wet or dry; straight or knotted; hydrophobic or hydrophilic), the storage condition of the suture, and whether or not it can be re-autoclaved.

Wound Breaking Strength It is the limit of tensile strength of a healing wound at which the wound edges gape or separate.

Straight-Pull Tensile Strength The suture strength varies for different knotting techniques. Straight-pull tensile strength refers to the linear breaking strength of the suture.

2.4 Size of Sutures

There are two classifications of suture size, one as per the United States Pharmacopeia (USP) and the other as per the European system. The USP method uses a complex relationship between diameter, tensile strength, and knot security, while the European system uses the diameter of the suture in millimeters.

Globally, USP is more commonly used. The commonly used suture size in ophthalmology ranges from 5-0 to 11-0 (Table 2.1) and is chosen depending on the structure to be sutured and the material used.

Table 2.1 Size of absorbable and nonabsorbable sutures

USP designation	Synthetic absorbable diameter (mm)	Nonabsorbable diameter (mm)
11-0		0.01
10-0	0.02	0.02
9-0	0.03	0.03
8-0	0.04	0.04
7-0	0.05	0.05
6-0	0.07	0.07
5-0	0.1	0.1
4-0	0.15	0.15
3-0	0.2	0.2
2-0	0.3	0.3
0	0.35	0.35
1	0.4	0.4
2	0.5	0.5
3	0.6	0.6
4	0.6	0.6
5	0.7	0.7
6		0.8

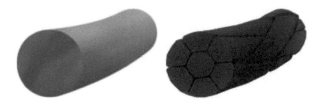

Fig. 2.1 Monofilament (single strand) and multifilament (multiple braided strands)

Monofilament Sutures These sutures have a single smooth strand, thus create less drag when passing through tissues, and resist harboring infections. The drawback with these sutures is that they have poor knot security as they crush and crimp easily, thus reducing the tensile strength.

Multifilament Sutures These sutures consist of several strands that are twisted together, which provide better tensile strength, flexibility, and pliability but increase drag on the tissues (Fig. 2.1).

Pseudo-monofilaments Some sutures may have a braided core within a smooth sleeve of extruded material.

2.5   Types of Sutures

Sutures can be classified as either absorbable or nonabsorbable depending on whether the body will naturally and gradually degrade or absorb the material.

Sutures have varied colors, and color of suture carries importance while working in a bloody field for easier identification and differentiation and while removing sutures.

2.5.1   Absorbable Sutures

Absorbable suture materials include the erstwhile natural catgut (made from the dried and treated connective tissue of cow or sheep intestines) and the newer synthetic sutures such as polylactic acid, polyglycolic acid, polydioxanone, and caprolactone. The polymer materials used in synthetic sutures are formulated on one or more of five cyclic monomers: glycolide, p-dioxanone, l-lactide, trimethylene carbonate, and ε-caprolactone.

These are broken down by proteolytic enzymatic degradation and hydrolysis (polyglycolic acid). The absorption process can range from 10 days to 8 weeks, depending on the material.

They are used to repair deeper tissues in layers or in patients who cannot return for suture removal. In both cases, they will hold the tissues together long enough to allow healing, but will disintegrate so that they do not leave foreign material

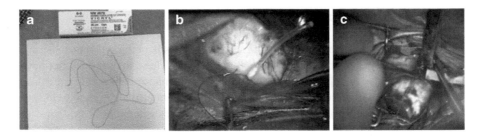

Fig. 2.2 (**a**) 6-0 Vicryl; (**b**) Ahmed glaucoma valve tube being anchored by Vicryl; (**c**) Vicryl for strabismus surgery

(temporary tissue support). There is an initial, transient foreign body reaction to the material, but after complete resorption only connective tissue remains. Sometimes, absorbable sutures can cause inflammation and be rejected by the body rather than absorbed.

- *Polyglactin*: Polyglactin 910 sutures (Vicryl®, Ethicon Inc.) are made from a copolymer of 90% glycolic acid and 10% lactic acid. The coated version (polyglactin 370 and calcium stearate) is the one available for ophthalmic use (Fig. 2.2), having less tissue drag despite being braided and mounted on spatulated or reverse-cutting needles.

  Absorption occurs through hydrolytic degradation. As Vicryl is slow-absorbing and braided, it must not be used for closure of any skin wounds exposed to the air, as it draws moisture from the healing tissue to the skin and allows microbial migration into the wound. This results in high reactivity to the contaminants, poor wound healing, and eventually infection.
- *Polyglycolic acid*: Polyglycolic acid sutures are made from braided or monofilament glycolic acid only, so their absorption is dependent on hydrolysis, an advantage when compared to enzymatic degradation, which tends to cause more inflammation. The tensile strength of both glycolic acid types will last for 2–3 weeks, but the material will remain in the tissue for about 2 or 3 months.
- *Polydioxanone (PDO):* This suture retains its tensile strength for up to 6 weeks, so it serves as a good option for suturing inner tissues requiring mechanical support, such as extraocular muscles, or for retaining an Ahmed glaucoma valve (AGV) or a Baerveldt glaucoma implant (BGI) in place, until the fibrous tissue grows through their holes and stabilizes them. The absorption occurs by hydrolysis, first as loss of tensile strength followed by loss of mass. Knots must be secured appropriately with additional throws, as PDO is monofilament.
- *Caprolactone:* Poly Glycolide Co-Caprolactone (PGCL) Sutures are synthetic monofilaments that absorb quickly into the body. PGCL Sutures are useful for short-term soft tissue approximation and/or ligation.

2.5.2 Nonabsorbable Sutures

Nonabsorbable sutures are made of special surgical grade silk or the synthetic materials such as polypropylene, polyester, or polyamide (nylon). These may or may not have coatings to enhance their performance characteristics. Nonabsorbable sutures are used either on skin wound closure, where the sutures can be removed after a few weeks, or in stressful internal environments where absorbable sutures will not hold up.

- *Silk*: Surgical grade silk is usually braided, pigmented, and degummed fibroin, with natural waxes removed and coated with several mixtures of waxes for smoothness (Fig. 2.3). It is considered a nonabsorbable suture since it retains its tensile strength for about 3–6 months, although residues of the suture may be found up to a couple of years later.
- *Polyamide/Nylon*: Polyamide is a relatively flexible monofilament suture that has high tensile strength, elasticity, and luster. It loses only about 10–15% of its tensile strength per year. The suture has low tissue drag, less memory, and good strength. It is ideal for suturing avascular, slow-healing tissues, such as the cornea (Fig. 2.4), with a very low chance of cutting through the tissue. It is also ideal for adjusting the curvature of the cornea in a relatively predictable manner or closing trabeculectomy flaps.
- *Polypropylene*: Polypropylene is also a monofilament suture that is capable of maintaining its tensile strength for extended periods of time. It is relatively rigid, so it can easily cheese-wire through sclera if handled improperly. It is the appropriate for scleral fixation of intraocular lens (Fig. 2.5), pupilloplasty, iridodialysis repair, brow lift, and correction of involutional ectropion.
- *Polyester*: Polyester is available for sutures in two forms: polytetrafluoroethylene (Gore-Tex) suture and polybutylate-coated braided polyester (Ethibond) suture. Polytetrafluoroethylene polyester suture has been found to give better results than polybutylate-coated braided polyester, for scleral buckling and as sling for frontalis suspension in bilateral congenital ptosis.

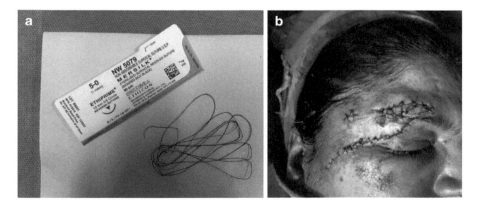

Fig. 2.3 (a) 5-0 silk; (b) skin suture with 5-0 silk

Fig. 2.4 (**a**) 10-0 nylon used for keratoplasty; (**b**) 9-0 nylon

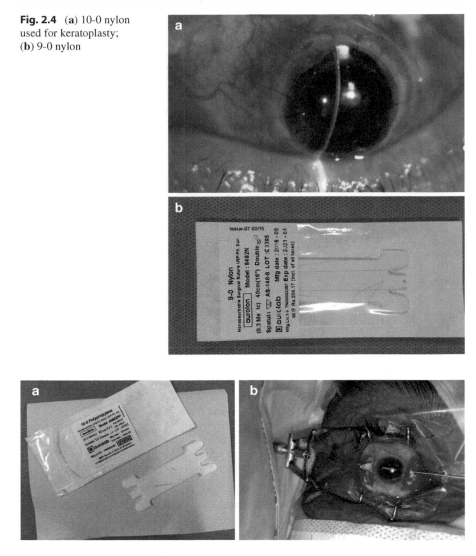

Fig. 2.5 (**a**) 10-0 polypropylene; (**b**) polypropylene being used for trans-scleral fixation of intra-ocular lens with the help of long 26G needle

Polyester sutures essentially never loose tensile strength and so are suitable for tying down canthal tendons or fixing scleral bands. Although the material is inert, it may become contaminated, causing occasional granulomas, or it can also erode through the conjunctiva with time. Therefore it is not a preferred suture for glaucoma implants.

Table 2.2 shows the commonly used sutures for various ophthalmic surgeries.

Table 2.2 Sutures used in common ophthalmic surgeries

Surgery	Sutures used
Pterygium	8-0 Vicryl 4-0 silk (traction suture)
Extra-/intracapsular cataract extraction	10-0 nylon
Trabeculectomy	5-0 silk (traction suture) 10-0/9-0 nylon 8-0 Vicryl
Glaucoma drainage device implantation	9-0 nylon/10–0 nylon 6-0 Vicryl (tube ligation) 8-0 Vicryl
Trans-scleral fixation of intraocular lens	10-0 polypropylene (double armed) 8-0 Vicryl
Scleral buckling	5-0 polyester 8-0 Vicryl 4-0 silk
Pars plana vitrectomy	7-0 Vicryl (double armed) 5-0 polypropylene
Keratoplasty	10-0 nylon
Ptosis surgery	4-0/5-0/6-0 silk 6-0 Vicryl 5-0 polypropylene (double armed)
Dacryocystorhinostomy	5-0 silk, 6-0 silk 6-0 Vicryl
Strabismus surgery	4-0 /5-0 silk (stay suture) 6-0 Vicryl (double armed) 8-0 Vicryl
Lid repair	5-0/4-0 silk 6-0 Vicryl
Open globe injury repair	10-0/ 9-0 nylon 5-0 polyester 8-0 Vicryl

2.5.3   Recent Innovations in Sutures

2.5.3.1 Drug-Eluting Sutures

Drug-eluting sutures have the potential to prevent postoperative infection and preclude issues with compliance that may result in the development of ulcers, endophthalmitis, and antibiotic resistance. Recently, an absorbable, ophthalmic-sized suture for sustained in vitro release of levofloxacin and inhibition of *S. epidermidis* has been developed using wet spinning technique. The suture is composed of poly(L-lactide) (PLLA) and polyethylene glycol (PEG) and levofloxacin. After implantation in the rat cornea, histology has shown it to be similar to commercially available nylon. Currently, drug-eluting sutures lack the required tensile strength, but the future holds promise.

2.6 Needles

The surgical needle allows the placement of the suture within the tissue, carrying the material through with minimal residual trauma. The needles are made of fine steel wire and drilled lengthwise.

The ideal surgical needle must be:

- Thin to minimize trauma
- Flexible enough to bend before breaking
- Rigid enough to resist distortion
- Sharp to penetrate tissue with minimal resistance
- Stable within the needle holder to allow for accurate placement

Parts of a Needle A suture needle has three parts: needle end, body, and point.

(a) *Needle ends:* Needles can be "eyed" or "eyeless/swaged."
  - "Eyed" needles have a hole at the suture side of the needle and need to be threaded with suture. These needles can be reused, but are not preferred as they are traumatic and unthread prematurely.
  - Swaged needles have the suture crimped within the needle and thus have markedly reduced risk of leakage along the suture line. These are less traumatic as single suture strand passes through the tissue.
(b) *Needle body and point*
  - Round body: These needles can either have sharp or blunt points. These pierce the tissues with minimal cutting and hence are used at sites where watertight closure is needed, e.g., conjunctival flap closure in trabeculectomy.
  - Triangular body: Needles with triangular-shaped bodies wherein each of the three edges is a cutting edge are also referred to as "cutting" needles. They are used to penetrate tough tissues and are ideal for suturing skin. A drawback of this needle is that it may pull out tissue during the creation of the needle track, which is just superficial to its tip.

    "Conventional" cutting needles have the cutting edge on the concave surface. "Reverse" cutting needles have their cutting surfaces on the convex surface, and there is a reduced risk of cutting through tissue. They are ideal for tough tissues. Reverse-cutting needles have more strength than conventional cutting needles. The suture canal, however, is deep to the needle tip. This makes the needle ideal for full thickness sutures through epidermis and skin. A drawback is that accidental perforations may result when partial thickness sutures are placed, a real drawback for suturing through the sclera since it may cut the choroid and/or cause suprachoroidal bleeding.

    Taper point is circular in cross section, with the cutting edge at the tip only, and therefore creating the smallest needle track of all the available needles. It is relatively atraumatic and is the preferred choice for iris and vascular repair. It is also useful for closing conjunctival advancements and bleb repairs when aqueous leaks are present. The drawback is the greater resistance to passing through the tissues, which can make the thinnest needles (e.g., 10-0 nylon) bend after a few passes.

The spatulated needle is the most versatile needle, with four to six cutting edges to the point, in cross section. It cuts at the sides and at the tip, parallel to the tissue plane in which it is passed through, avoiding any accidental perforations. It provides the surgeon with proprioceptive feedback when it is passed through the parallel-stacked fibers of both the cornea and sclera. Figure 2.6 shows the notations used for needle cross section on the suture packs.

(c) *Needle curvature*
- Straight needles: This needle is designed to be used without the aid of instruments (by hand). It is used when tissue is easily accessible, e.g., for skin closure or microsurgical procedures like vessel repair.
- Half-curved: Also known as Ski; used to suture using laparoscopic technique.
- Half curved at both ends of a straight segment (Canoe).
- 1/4 circle: This needle has a shallow curvature thus ideal for easily accessible convex surfaces. Typically used for ophthalmic and microsurgical procedures (Fig. 2.7).
- 3/8 circle: Most commonly used for large and superficial wounds. Not preferable for deep cavities due to large arc of manipulation.
- 1/2 circle: This needle is good for confined locations, but the only difficulty is need for more pronation and supination of wrists.
- 5/8 circle: This needle is ideal for deep, confined holes and can be used by rotating the wrist with little to no lateral movement.
- Compound curve.

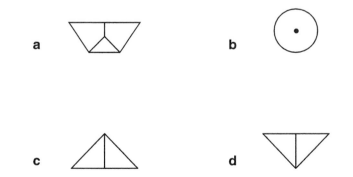

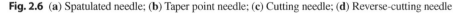

Fig. 2.6 (**a**) Spatulated needle; (**b**) Taper point needle; (**c**) Cutting needle; (**d**) Reverse-cutting needle

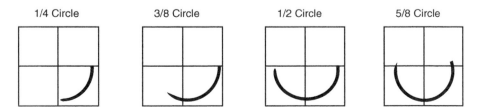

Fig. 2.7 Commonly used needle curvatures

Fig. 2.8 (**a**) Single-armed curved suture; (**b**) double-armed curved suture; (**c**) double-armed (one straight, one curved) suture; (**d**) double-armed straight suture

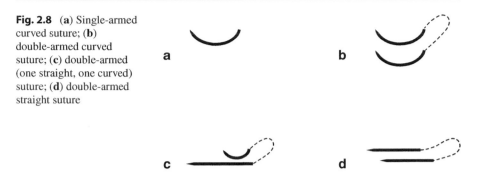

Figure 2.8 shows the notations used for curvature and type of needle on the suture packs.

2.6.1 Points to Remember

- Suture material should be chosen keeping in mind the tissue type, risk of infection, and surgeon's personal preferences. The smallest suture material that properly holds tissues should be used.
- The free needles having an eye at the proximal end are sometimes useful in passing the other end of suture (not having needle) from the same side of tissues to form a loop. For example, in LPS resection surgery, the other end of 6-0 Prolene suture is passed through the LPS muscle.
- Do not hold the monofilament suture with needle holder as it reduces the tensile strength by ~50%.
- Hold the needle at proximal 1/3–2/3 junction.
- Never hold the needle from its swaged end. The suture and needle attachment weakens.
- Sutures are presterilized with gamma radiation, but if they need to be re-sterilized, then immerse them in 10% povidone-iodine solution for 10 min, and then rinse thoroughly with saline.

Suggested Readings

1. Albis-Donado O, Bhartiya S, Casale-Vargas G. Sutures and needles in ophthalmology. In: Ichhpujani P, Spaeth GL, Yanoff M, editors. Expert techniques in ophthalmic surgery. 1st ed. Vijayawada: Jaypee Brothers Medical Publisher; 2015. p. 25–9.
2. Kashiwabuchi F, Parikh KS, Omiadze R, et al. Development of absorbable, antibiotic-eluting sutures for ophthalmic surgery. Transl Vis Sci Technol. 2017;6(1):1.

Basics of Surgical Instruments

3

Manpreet Singh, Manpreet Kaur, Natasha Gautam, and Sonam Yangzes

3.1 Definition of a Surgical Instrument

A surgical instrument is a specially designed tool or device which is used to perform or facilitate a few specific actions during a surgical procedure or operation. The use of a specially designed surgical instrument helps in achieving the best possible outcome with efficiency and minimum complications.

An instrument can have a specific medical (diagnostic) or surgical (therapeutic) role. Each surgical instrument is used to carry out the desired effects such as *holding* (forceps, clamps, and needle holders) and *modifying biological tissue* (cutting, stretching, and breaking) or *to provide access* for viewing the deeper tissues (retractors, suction). The surgical instruments are broadly divided into "sharps" and "blunts."

- *Sharps:* These include scissors, blades, knives, trocars, needles, trephines, rongeurs, and razor fragments.
- *Blunts:* These include speculum, needle holders, hemostatic clamps, retractors, spatulas, loops, cannulas, hooks, and forceps.

M. Singh (✉)
Oculoplastics Services, Department of Ophthalmology, Advanced Eye Centre, Post Graduate Institute of Medical Education and Research (PGIMER), Chandigarh, India

M. Kaur · N. Gautam
Glaucoma Services, Department of Ophthalmology, Advanced Eye Centre, Post Graduate Institute of Medical Education and Research (PGIMER), Chandigarh, India

S. Yangzes
Cataract and Refractive Services, Department of Ophthalmology, Advanced Eye Centre, Post Graduate Institute of Medical Education and Research (PGIMER), Chandigarh, India

© Springer Nature Singapore Pte Ltd. 2019
P. Ichhpujani, M. Singh (eds.), *Ophthalmic Instruments and Surgical Tools*,
Current Practices in Ophthalmology,
https://doi.org/10.1007/978-981-13-7673-3_3

For a systematic description of a surgical instrument, a single preset pattern is followed everywhere and in our book.

3.2   Instrument Nomenclature

It is one of the essential parts of the instrument description as the instrument name acknowledges its inventor and helps in building an efficient intraoperative understanding between the surgeon and assistant about the need of a specific type of instrument for a specific surgical step.

The nomenclature of an instrument follows certain patterns – the name of its inventor/doctor, the function it performs (forceps, scissors, retractors, clamps, etc.), its appearance (cat's paw, mosquito forceps, ribbon retractors, etc.), or a scientific name related to the surgery (ptosis clamp, chalazion clamp and curette, etc.). One should understand the rationale behind the instrument nomenclature for a better understanding of its action and nature.

Inside an operation theatre, the surgical instruments constitute the essential part of the surgeon's armamentarium. Due to the large number and variety of surgical instruments in different specialties of ophthalmology, the residents and fellows find it challenging to remember the names and appreciate the subtle differences of action from each other and the uses of each surgical instrument. Moreover, the fineness of the instrument tips amplifies the challenge to accurately identify one on-trolley while assisting and during the practical examinations. This makes one feel intimidated to handle the instruments correctly. Keeping this in mind, we have tried to describe the surgical instruments in a single, simple, preset pattern for easier identification and description.

3.3   General Functions of Surgical Instruments

- *Holding or grasping of tissue*: This function is performed by the forceps, holders, clamps, etc.
- *Cutting, incising, punching, or breaking:* This specific action is executed by scissors, blades, knives, chisels, awls, rongeur, punches, etc.
- *Retraction or separation:* The retraction is provided by speculums, hooks, or retractors.
- *Aspiration, injection, draining, or irrigation:* Suction tips, needles, catheters, cannulas, syringes, drains, etc. can be used to evacuate the blood/ fluid/pus from the operative field without disturbing the ongoing process.
- *Probing and dilatation*: To traverse a tubular path and to widen a small opening, probes, stylet, dilators, etc. are required.
- *Cautery or hemostasis:* To perform this action, a fire-heated or electricity-heated instrument is used especially working in a vascular region.
- *Apposition*: This specific feature is of tissue glues, sutures, stickers, staplers, etc.

3.4   Anatomical Description of a Surgical Instrument

Handle of an instrument: This is the main part of the instrument by which it is held in the hand of an operating surgeon or an assistant (Fig. 3.1). The handles can be ring handles, interlocked leaf handles (most common in ophthalmology), or grooved handle variety.

Blade types: Depending upon the tip and the cutting edge of the two blades of a scissor, these are classified as *sharp-sharp* (both tips are sharp), *blunt-blunt, sharp-blunt* (one tip is sharp, and other is blunt), *blunt with bevel*, fine-tip sharp, fine-tip blunt, etc. (Fig. 3.2).

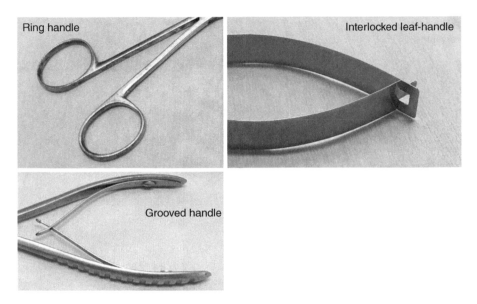

Fig. 3.1 Types of instrument handles

Fig. 3.2 Types of instrument blades

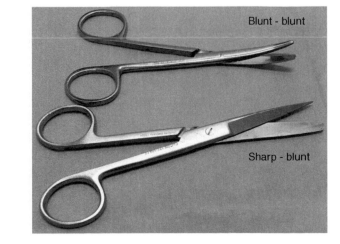

Blade curvature types: This is a simple description of the blades in an open or closed position which can be *straight, curved, angled-on-flat, bayonet-shaped,* etc. (Fig. 3.3).

Joint types: This is a critical part of an instrument as far as its manufacturing, functioning, and cleaning are concerned. These are categorized as *box lock, lap joint,* and *double action joint* types (Fig. 3.4).

Position retaining system: This part of the instrument constitutes a system which retains its original position (Fig. 3.5). Mainly a lock or spring keeps the business end of the instrument in the desired position. These systems are *double leaf spring, ratchet lock, single or double spring, with roller or ball and socket joint,* etc.

Fig. 3.3 Types of blade curvatures

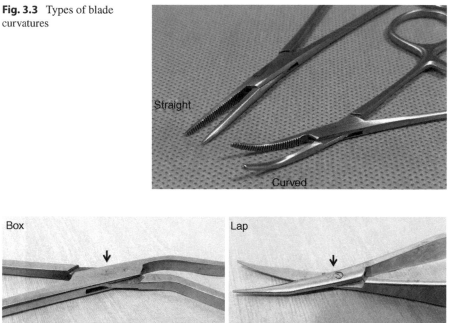

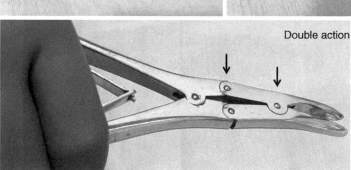

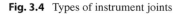

Fig. 3.4 Types of instrument joints

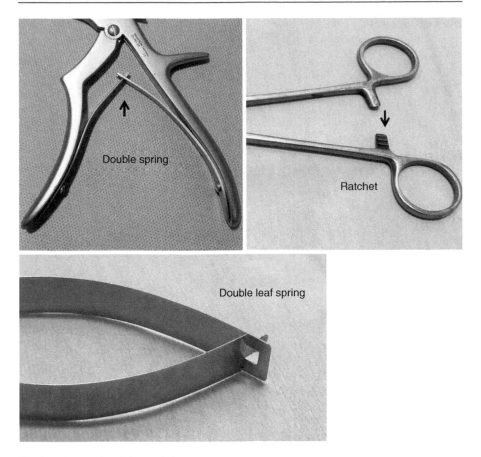

Fig. 3.5 Types of position retaining systems

Guide pins: These pins are present on the inner surface of one limb of forceps which is guided into a locating hole on the opposite limb of forceps (Fig. 3.6). This is to ensure the accuracy of the jaws' mating. According to British Standards, the guide pin shall be tapered to facilitate entry into the locating hole and shall not protrude from the hole when the jaws are closed. When a surgeon closes the forceps with more force than required, the guide pin protrudes and pokes the finger pulp of surgeon, pointing at reducing the pressure over the limbs of forceps. This may also become a source of glove puncture.

3.5   Instrument Materials

- *Stainless steel (SS):* It is the most commonly used material/alloy for manufacturing surgical instruments (Fig. 3.7a) due to its strength, corrosion resistance, and affordability. The amount of chromium (12–14%) added to this alloy

Fig. 3.6 Guide pins

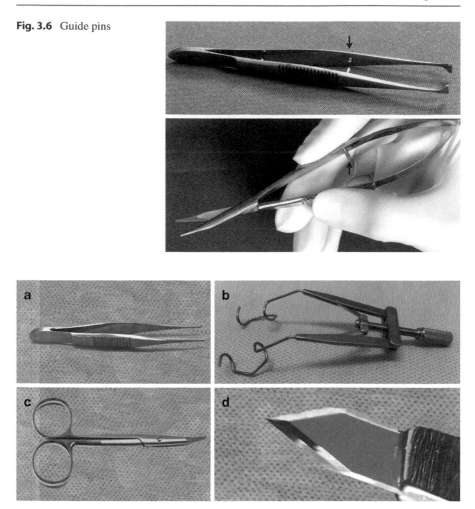

Fig. 3.7 Instrument materials; (**a**) Stainless Steel; (**b**) Titanium; (**c**) Tungsten carbide; (**d**) Diamond

makes it corrosion-resistant, rather than its "stainless" label, which is a misnomer. The minimum carbon content of the steel (0.17–0.25%) still renders it "at risk" for rusting and corrosion. Generally, two variants of SS are used to manufacture ophthalmic surgical instruments – *austenitic* (series 300) and *martensitic* (series 400).

The austenitic variety is nonmagnetic, non-heat-treated, lower in carbon content, and robust; hence it is used in the manufacturing of instruments like speculums, calipers, retractors, etc. On the other hand, the martensitic steel which is heat-treated, strong, and magnetic is used to fabricate scissors, curettes, cutters, trephines, needle holders, etc. The protective "passive" layer over the SS instruments can provide durability and resist corrosion. Mechanical trauma causing pitting, scratches, abrasions, or micro-abrasions accelerates the corrosion process. The required strength, flexibility, and malleability are the targets of all instrument manufacturing companies which provide these efficiently designed instruments.

- *Titanium (Ti):* As compared to SS, titanium is lighter, harder, and stronger but costlier. Its biocompatibility, corrosion-resistance, nonmagnetic, and rustproof properties make it ideal to use for ophthalmic surgical instruments which need fine manipulations and heavy turnover (Fig. 3.7b). The rigidity of the element is exploited to make very fine instruments having delicate teeth or tips. Moreover, the light reflections working under the microscope are reduced, and these instruments can be used safely for the image-guided surgeries. Its medical grade alloy (grade 23) is composed of aluminum (4%) and vanadium (4%). The surface of titanium forms an inert or negatively charged oxide film which is protective for ionic degradation and corrosion. Bone plates, screws, wires, artificial joints, prosthesis, dentistry items, rods, etc. are made up of titanium due to its excellent biocompatibility.
- *Tungsten carbide (TC):* This alloy contains carbon and tungsten in equal parts and is compressed to form surgical instruments (Fig. 3.7c) and cutting tools like drills and burrs (high-speed tools). It can withstand high degrees of temperature and pressure and is twice stiffer than SS. Heavy-duty surgical instruments like needle holders, scissors, wire tighteners, pliers, etc. are made up of TC. The higher cost makes it less affordable to be used in surgical instruments, though they last four to five times longer than its stainless steel counterparts.
- *Diamond:* Diamond, by virtue of its durability and sharpness, is used to make keratomes (Fig. 3.7d) (for cataract or anterior segment surgeries) and retinal diamond-dusted brushes. As the material itself is very expensive, it demands special attention and care.
- *Fiber optics:* This material is used for transmitting the light in the most efficient way from the source to the target organ. Laser indirect ophthalmoscope (LIO), endolights for retinal surgeries, and nasal endoscopes are few examples which use these filaments working on the basis of total internal reflection. The wires containing these optical fibers are rendered fragile and need gentle and careful handling. Acute bending of wires and putting heavy weights over these crush the sensitive optical filaments. Plasma sterilization is the desirable way to prepare these wires for intraoperative use.

3.6   Stages of Instrument Fabrication

- *Forging:* In this process, the precut stainless steel bars are compressed and shaped under tons of weight. Forging can be done either after heating SS bars at very high temperatures (hot forging) or normal temperature (cold forging).
- *Milling and turning:* The basic shape of forceps, locks, jaws, and ratchets is formed during this stage.
- *Assembly:* The male-female or similar parts of an instrument are joined together and assembled at this stage.

- *Filing and grinding:* This step requires great skill, and the fineness of the work performed at this step finalizes the shape of an instrument.
- *Heat treatment:* This varies according to the chosen instrument material (stainless steel, titanium, etc.). During this step, the instrument is subjected to very high temperatures followed by cooling to make it sturdy enough to withstand the rigors of usage and autoclaving process.
- *Fitting and polishing:* The fine-tuning of shape and aesthetic look to the instrument is given at this step. Hence, it is the most important step for the scissors and fine-toothed instruments used in routine ophthalmic surgeries.
- *Final inspection under magnification:* Handheld or table-mounted magnifiers are used to inspect the final finishing of the product with focus on the business end.

Suggested Reading

1. Kapczynski H. An introduction to KMedic certified instruments in 'A manual of surgical instruments 101'. 1997. pp. A4–A14.

Anterior Segment Surgery Instruments

4

Sahil Thakur, Natasha Gautam Seth, Monika Balyan, and Parul Ichhpujani

4.1 Introduction

Surgical instruments are the proverbial "workhorse" of the ophthalmic surgeons. The instruments described in this chapter are some of the most commonly encountered by those dealing with ocular surgery. Although not always recognized, a proper understanding of surgical instruments plays a vital role in good surgical patient outcomes. Incorrect handling and use of surgical instruments can reduce precision and increase fatigue. Recent literature shows that surgeons performing minimally invasive surgery (MIS) when compared with surgeons performing open surgery were significantly more likely to experience pain in the neck, arm, shoulder, hands, and legs and experience higher odds of fatigue and numbness [1]. Factors like instrument ergonomics, surgeon posture, and surgery duration have been correlated to these symptoms. It is unfortunate that 59–99% of surgeons are unaware of the ergonomic recommendations of their institutions and usually none receive mandatory ergonomic training [1, 2].

Proper knowledge about surgical instruments and appropriate use can significantly improve patient outcomes. This knowledge can also improve surgeon ergonomics and decrease strain. Thus this chapter tries to fill in that lacuna between "routine" and

S. Thakur (⊠)
Department of Ocular Epidemiology, Singapore Eye Research Institute, Singapore

N. G. Seth
Glaucoma Services, Department of Ophthalmology, Advanced Eye Centre, Post Graduate Institute of Medical Education and Research (PGIMER), Chandigarh, India

M. Balyan
Cataract and Refractive Services, Department of Ophthalmology, Advanced Eye Centre, Post Graduate Institute of Medical Education and Research (PGIMER), Chandigarh, India

P. Ichhpujani
Glaucoma Services, Government Medical College and Hospital, Chandigarh, India

© Springer Nature Singapore Pte Ltd. 2019
P. Ichhpujani, M. Singh (eds.), *Ophthalmic Instruments and Surgical Tools*,
Current Practices in Ophthalmology,
https://doi.org/10.1007/978-981-13-7673-3_4

"ideal" use of these anterior segment surgery instruments. Some of the instruments might be covered again in the subsequent chapters, as some overlap is unavoidable.

4.2 The Speculums

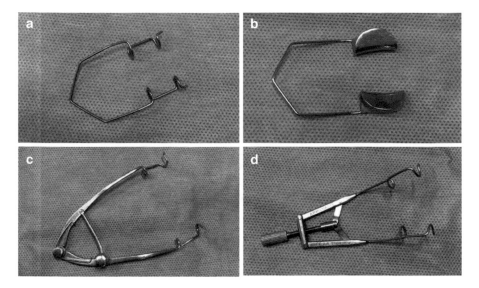

Fig. 4.1 (**a**) Barraquer Eye Speculum (Fenestrated Blade); (**b**) Barraquer Eye Speculum (Solid Blade); (**c**) Weiss Eye Speculum; (**d**) self-retaining universal eye speculum

Key Points
- A speculum consists of two limbs with adjustable/nonadjustable mechanism, joined at one end and open/closed/wired/solid blades at the open end.
- The adjustable variety contains a guard/locking mechanism with a screw by which the width of the open end of speculum can be adjusted. The nonadjustable variety usually has a spring mechanism.
- Universal: Can be used for both the eyes.
- Lightweight: Avoids direct pressure on the globe.
- The speculums can be broadly subdivided into adjustable and nonadjustable speculums (Fig. 4.1):
  - *Adjustable:* Lieberman, Saunders, Murdoch, Mellinger, Knapp, Lancaster, Williams, Castroviejo
  - *Nonadjustable:* Wire speculum (Barraquer, Kratz-Barraquer, Sauer, Alfonso)
  - *Pediatric speculums:* Weiss, Sauer, Cook, Alfonso, Barraquer Pediatric Speculum

Instrument Handling After cleaning the surgical eye field and application of eye drape, the drape is cut in the center, and the speculum is inserted in such a way that the joint end of the speculum is placed temporally and the open end with blades faces nasally retracting both the upper and lower lid. The upper blades are inserted first retracting the upper lid so that the lashes do not interfere with the surgical field, followed by retraction of lower lid and insertion of lower blades. The Barraquer Eye Speculum is used widely as it keeps both the eyelid margin and eyelashes out of the operative field.

Uses
The speculums are used to retract the lids during:

- Intraocular surgery: cataract surgery, glaucoma filtration surgery, glaucoma drainage device, etc.
- Extraocular surgery: squint surgery, pterygium excision, oculoplasty surgeries (enucleation/evisceration)
- Examination of a patient with blepharospasm
- Slit lamp procedures: removal of the corneal foreign body, releasable suture removal/injection of 5-fluorouracil after glaucoma filtration surgery in uncooperative patients
- Examination of children suspected of open/closed globe injury in the outpatient department
- Can be used to perform fundus examination using +20D lens and mobile devices
- Can be used in patients with difficulty in keeping the lid open while ocular imaging procedures like OCT and biometry
- Laser procedures like a prophylactic laser of peripheral retinal breaks
- Intraocular injections like intravitreal anti-VEGF and antibiotics in endophthalmitis

Recent Innovations Innovative products like disposable lid speculum with a drape (Li Drape®, Hakko Co., Ltd., Nagano, Japan) have been developed for simple and complete draping of the eyelashes and eyelids to ensure an appropriate surgical field. The drape has also been demonstrated to decrease surgical field contamination in cataract surgery patients successfully [3].

4.3   The Forceps

Key Features
- Forceps are two bladed instruments with a handle used to grasp/compress the tissues while performing surgery. Most of the ophthalmic forceps come under the category of tissue/thumb forceps because they are operated by compression between thumb and forefinger.
- The forceps consist of three principal parts: the tip, the shaft, and the handle.
  - *Handle:* It is the part where the instrument is being handled/gripped by the surgeon. It can have grooves to facilitate the grip, or there can be a handle with holes in it. It increases the working area and helps in easy manipulation in the surgical field. The handle can be flat that allows good manual grip but requires significant hand, wrist, or forearm movements. Round handles allow better "micro" control of the tip with minimum movement. Cross action handles can open/close tips by putting and releasing pressure and offer significant micro control.
  - *Shaft:* This part connects the handle with the tip. The shaft may be straight (direct access), curved (restricted access), angled (access at an angle), Colibri (better tip visualization), cross action (maximum tip opening with a small incision), or designed for a specific purpose (lens forceps).
  - *Tip:* This is the working end of the forceps. The tip may be plain (general purpose like removing cilia), serrated (atraumatic grasping of tissues), platform (for tying, holding, and removing sutures), notched (grasping and holding tissues, tubes, needles, etc.), or toothed. The toothed forceps can have different types of alignments: (a) opposing type, flat opposing surface, less traumatic but less grasp than other variants like Pierse Hoskins Forceps; (b) interdigitating type: usually have one into two patterns, i.e., one shaft has one tooth, and the opposing shaft has two teeth at the tip so that they snugly fit into each other; (c) tooth at right angles, the teeth are aligned at right angles, e.g., Bishop-Harmon forceps; and (d) forward angled tooth, the teeth are angulated to facilitate grasp and manipulation, e.g., Castroviejo forceps (Table 4.1).

Uses
Some of the commonly used forceps are described overleaf in Table 4.2 (Fig. 4.2).

Table 4.1 Ophthalmic subspecialties and common forceps

Type of surgeries	Commonly used forceps
Routine	Beer Cilia Forceps, Barraquer Cilia Forceps, Drews Forceps, Gradle Forceps
Lid and oculoplastic surgeries	Adson, Jewelers, Chalazion Clamp, artery/hemostatic forceps, Berke Ptosis Clamp, Putterman Forceps
Squint surgeries	Moorfields Forceps, superior rectus-holding forceps, globe fixation forceps
Conjunctiva	Moorfields Forceps, Pierse Hoskins Forceps, plain forceps, Bishop-Harmon Tissue Forceps
Cornea and refractive surgery	Colibri, Carlson DSEK graft, corneal flap forceps in LASIK
Sclera	Colibri, plain forceps
Suturing	McPherson, Kelman-McPherson, Harm's tying, Castroviejo, Bishop-Harmon, plain forceps
Iris	Iris forceps
Lens	Utrata capsulorhexis, Arruga capsule-holding forceps, IOL implantation forceps (Neuhann/Fechner/Doden/Shepard/Tenner)
Retina	Lander's vitrectomy lens forceps, ILM peeling, end grasping forceps

Table 4.2 Commonly used forceps in ocular surgery

Forceps	Key features	Uses
Non-toothed/smooth tip		
Plain forceps	• Straight forceps • Grooved handle • Tips are smooth but vertically/horizontally serrated	• Used where atraumatic handling of tissues is required • Hold scleral flap during glaucoma filtration procedure • Hold nasal/lacrimal mucosal flaps during DCR • Suture tying forceps
Moorfields Forceps	• Stout and straight • Grooves in handle • A small opening with the guard in handle in some • Horizontal serrations at the stout tip with oval serration free zone in it	• Easy handling of slippery conjunctiva during strabismus surgeries
McPherson	• Fine forceps with three-round fenestrations in both limbs of handle • Straight, smooth tipped with triangular-shaped opposing edges	• Used in fine suturing like 10-0 nylon in keratoplasty and trabeculectomy
Kelman-McPherson	• Fine forceps with three-round fenestrations in both limbs of handle • Guard • Angled limbs (shaft)	• Used in fine suturing like 10-0 nylon in keratoplasty and trabeculectomy • Holding the optic of IOL while IOL insertion in Phaco/ECCE
Harms tying	• Fine forceps	• Used in fine suturing like 10-0 nylon in keratoplasty and trabeculectomy
Beer Cilia Forceps	• Small, stout forceps with grooved handle • Blunt and flat ends	• Epilate cilia in trichiasis

(continued)

Table 4.2 (continued)

Forceps	Key features	Uses
Tooth forceps		
Adson forceps	• Straight forceps • Grooved handle • Tooth at right angles	• Hold skin during lid and oculoplastic surgeries
Globe fixation forceps	• Grooved handle • Stout shaft and tip • Forward angled 2 × 3 or 3 × 4 tooth at the tip	• Applied near the limbus to hold the conjunctiva and Tenon firmly during • Forced duction test • Fix the eyeball during surgery
Pierse Hoskins Forceps	• Three-round fenestrations in both limbs of handle • Tips have a concavity facing each other with the flat opposing surface	• Less traumatic but less firm grasp than other tooth forceps • Hold conjunctiva and muscle during squint surgeries
Superior rectus-holding forceps	• Also known as Dastoor Forceps • Grooved handle • Hole with guard • S-shaped double curve near the tip • 1 × 2 tooth	• Used to hold the superior rectus tendon while passing bridle suture beneath it • Traction suture in various surgeries, e.g., extra capsular cataract extraction, glaucoma filtration surgery
Colibri forceps	• Italic word, meaning bird • Grooved handle • Flat platform • Angulated/curved shaft • Straight tip with fine tooth 1 × 2	• Ideal for holding cornea/sclera edge while suturing in • Open globe injury repair • Keratoplasty • Glaucoma filtration surgery *Double Colibri forceps* • Each side of the tip is horse shoe-shaped with interdigitating fine teeth at both sides to have a better grip of edges of donor and host cornea during keratoplasty
Lim's forceps	• Grooved handle • Guard • Flat shaft adjoining handle which is angled in front adjoining the tip • Straight tip with fine tooth 1 × 2	• Corneoscleral forceps used to hold cornea/sclera edge while suturing in • Open globe injury repair • Keratoplasty • Glaucoma filtration surgery
Bishop-Harmon Tissue Forceps	• Three-round fenestrations in both limbs of handle • Straight/curved shaft • 2 × 1 tooth aligned at right angles to each other	• The commonly used instrument in the lid and oculoplastic surgeries for holding tissues
Castroviejo suturing forceps	• Grooved handle • Straight-tipped • 2 × 1 tooth aligned at forwarding angles to each other	• Tissue holding forceps with forward angle helping in easy manipulation

Table 4.2 (continued)

Forceps	Key features	Uses
Utility forceps		
Chalazion clamp	• It has two limbs that can be clamped with the help of a screw • One limb is flat, while other is like a small circular ring; the flat side is applied toward the skin and ring toward the conjunctival side	• Chalazion excision, maintains hemostasis, adequate exposure
Entropion clamp	• It has two limbs, one looks like a D-shaped plate and other is a U-shaped rim that can be closed with a screw • The handle is kept toward the temporal side, plate toward conjunctiva, and rim on the skin side • Self-retaining	• Used for entropion/ectropion surgery
Artery/ hemostatic forceps	• Blunt tipped, stout forceps in a scissorlike configuration • Lock at the ring end • X-shaped hinge • Multiple serrations at the tip • Large, medium, and small (mosquito artery forceps) size • Straight and curved forceps	• Hold traction/stay sutures in oculoplastic and glaucoma surgeries • Catch bleeders in oculoplasty surgeries • In place of sponge holder while draping • To hold gauze pieces while packing the socket after evisceration

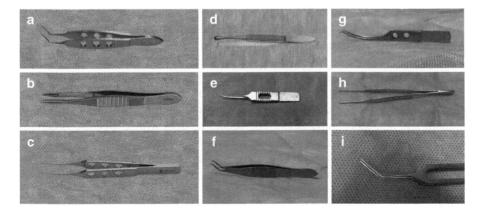

Fig. 4.2 (**a**) Kelman-McPherson Forceps; (**b**) Moorfields Forceps; (**c**) Pierse Hoskins Forceps; (**d**) Beer Cilia Forceps; (**e**) Harms forceps; (**f**) Dastoor superior rectus-holding forceps; (**g**): Lim's forceps; (**h**) globe fixation forceps; (**i**) Utrata's capsule-holding forceps

4.4   The Needle Holders

Key Features
- The needle holders consist of four principal parts: the tip, the jaws, the hinge, and the handle.
  - *Handle*: It is the part where the instrument is being handled/gripped by the surgeon. The handle can be flat that allows good manual grip but requires significant hand, wrist, or forearm movements. Round handles allow better "micro" control of the tip with minimum movement. Catch/lock mechanism handles can be used to lock the jaws in the closed position to facilitate securing of the needle during suturing.
  - *Jaws*: The jaws of these needle holders can be either straight or curved, but are short, sturdy, and delicate with flat inner platforms.
  - *Tip*: This is the working end of the needle holder. The tip may be fine (corneal sutures), standard (general purpose like cataract/trabeculectomy), or heavy (for larger sutures used in strabismus or lid surgery).
  - The needle holders can be broadly subdivided into locking and non-locking needle holders
    - *Locking*: Kalt Needle Holder, McPherson Locking Needle Holder, Arruga's Needle Holder, Steven's Needle Holder, Silcock's Needle Holder
    - *Non-locking*: Barraquer Needle Holder, Castroviejo Needle Holder

Instrument Handling   The handles of the needle holder are kept long to provide increased maneuverability while passing through delicate ocular structures. It also helps in providing desired holding pressure at the jaws with minimum force at handles. The flat inner surface of jaws prevents needle deformation. Generally, the needle should be held at the 2/3–1/3 junction from needle tip or 1/3 needle length from the swaged end. The spatulated needles have a rectangular cross section which keeps the needle stable and prevents its rotation. On the contrary, the swaged end and a round-body needle have a circular cross section which can lead to rotation of the needle. Excessive force over the swaged end of a suture can lead to its damage, causing suture loosening, detachment, or breakage. The handles of the needle holder should preferably be without lock while operating under a microscope, to have smooth and non-jerky movements. The needle holders with a lock are generally used by oculoplastic surgeons while operating with a magnifying loupe or the naked eye. Before sterilization, the joint of a needle holder should be properly cleaned for its smooth jaw movements.

Uses
- Can hold the body of a needle for passing it through tissues
- Commonly used to make a needle cystitome of 26-gauge needle tip
- Can be used to hold the suture while tying the knots
- Can be used to hold soft tissue like conjunctiva (Table 4.3, Fig. 4.3)

Table 4.3 Commonly used needle holders in ocular surgery

Needle holder	Key features	Uses
Non-locking		
Barraquer Needle Holder	• Spring-based • Round, cross-serrated grip • Usually has curved delicate jaws with serrations and blunt tips	• Used for holding small needles during microsurgery
Castroviejo Needle Holder	• Spring-based • Smooth jaws • Flat-serrated handles • The locking mechanism is also available in some models	• Used for holding small needles during microsurgery
Locking		
Kalt Needle Holder	• Multipurpose instrument • Flat handle but triangular design with thumb release • Delicate and cross-serrated jaws	• Used in fine suturing in oculoplasty procedures

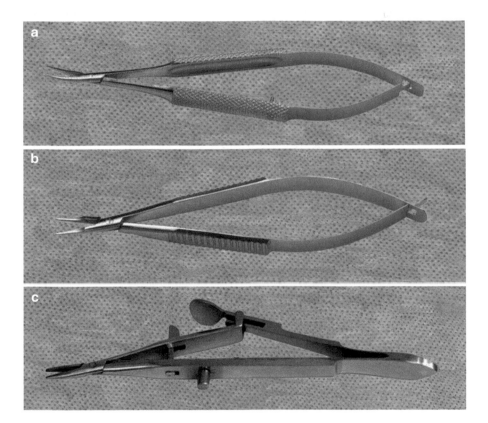

Fig. 4.3 (**a**) Barraquer Needle Holder; (**b**) Castroviejo Needle Holder; (**c**) Kalt locking needle holder

4.5   The Scissors

Key Features
- The scissors consist of four principal parts. The tip, the jaws, the hinge, and the handle.
  - *Handle*: It is the part where the instrument is being handled/gripped by the surgeon. The handle can be spring-based (offers good manual grip with excellent tip control, e.g., Vannas Scissors), bow-/ribbon-based (traditional design, good utility scissors for extra ocular application, require significant wrist/hand movement, e.g., Stevens Tenotomy Scissors), or hinge-based (blades close when handle is squeezed, used for iris excision, e.g., De Wecker Scissors).
  - *Jaws*: The jaws of scissors can be either straight, curved, or angled.
- *Tip*: This is the working end of the scissors. The tip may be sharp/pointed (can pierce as well as cut) or rounded (for only cutting).

Instrument Handling   The scissor points are extremely delicate and the tips should never be touched. All scissors, needle holders, and fine forceps should have their tips protected. The protectors must cover the whole blade or jaws of the instrument in order to protect the instrument edge and to prevent accidental injuries while sterilization. Scissors should only be used for their intended cutting purpose. Do not use them for prying, screwing, scraping, or pounding. It is vital to always cut away from your body in small, regular strokes. Often it is easier to cut from right to left when you are right-handed and from left to right when left-handed. Always visualize the tissue in between the cutting edge as it is easy to miss the intended structure if the instrument is used in a rushed manner. It is advisable to use scissors with your wrist held in a neutral position and not bent at awkward angles or positions.

Uses   Some of the commonly used scissors are described overleaf in Table 4.4 (Fig. 4.4).

Table 4.4 Commonly used scissors in ocular surgery

Scissors	Key features	Uses
Castroviejo Corneal Scissors	• Spring action • Can be straight, curved, or angled	• Used in keratoplasty, fine cutting, and suture division
Iris scissors	• Very light and delicate with sharp points • Can be straight or curved	• Cutting the iris
Stevens Tenotomy Scissors	• Ribbon type • Long handles, with a wide variety of tips available	• Delicate dissection and separation of tissues • Used to create tissue planes for implantation of devices like glaucoma drainage devices, scleral bands, etc.
Westcott Tenotomy Scissors	• Fine scissors with a spring mechanism	• Delicate dissection and cutting
Vannas Scissors	• Sharp tip scissors with a spring mechanism • Can be straight, curved, or angled	• Delicate cutting like iris abscission, capsulotomy, etc.
De Wecker Scissors	• Fine scissors with right-angled blades • Blades kept in V-shape due to spring action	• Used to perform iridectomy, iridotomy, and iris abscission
Enucleation Scissors	• Large, strong scissors • Curved blades • Ribbon type	• Used to cut the optic nerve during enucleation

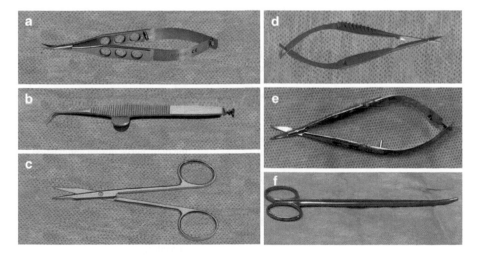

Fig. 4.4 (**a**) Westcott Tenotomy Scissor; (**b**) De Wecker Scissors; (**c**) Stevens Tenotomy Scissors; (**d**) Vannas Scissors; (**e**) Corneoscleral Scissors; (**f**) Enucleation Scissors

4.6 Miscellaneous

Some of the commonly used instruments are described briefly below in Table 4.5 (Figs. 4.5, 4.6, 4.7, 4.8, 4.9, 4.10, 4.11, and 4.12).

4.6.1 Recent Innovations and the Future

Surgical instruments are going to see much customization shortly. With a focus on ergonomics and personal preference, 3D printed instruments will be soon available catering to individual motion preference. With the ability of robotics and advanced gyroscopic sensors being harnessed for surgical manoeuvers, it will be able to account for human limitations like physiological tremors [4, 5]. Till those times become a reality, we can ensure that we keep our knowledge updated and our "instruments" sharp and ready.

Table 4.5 Commonly used other instruments in anterior segment surgeries

Instrument	Key features	Uses
Castroviejo callipers	• Dividers like instrument with one fixed arm that is attached to a graduated scale in millimeters and another movable arm	• Take measurements during squint, ptosis, pterygium, scleral buckling, and corneal surgeries
Muscles hooks		
Jameson Muscle Hook	• Straight shaft • 6 mm hook with a bulbous tip	• Retrieving the rectus muscles at their insertion sites with minimal distortion
Stevens muscle/ Tenotomy Hook	• Angled tip with a 4 mm blunt tip	• Retracting of ocular muscles during squint surgery
Knives/blades		
Keratomes	• Sharp angled/straight/curved/pointed/arrow shaped blades • Available in various sizes and shapes, e.g., 15^0 blades, 2.8 mm, 2.2 mm	• Used to make valvular corneal incisions of various dimension and depths
Spatulas/spoons/curettes		
Enucleation spoon	• Also called optic nerve guide • U shaped instrument	• Central groove is used to engage the optic nerve during enucleation procedure
Evisceration spatula	• Rectangular blade with slightly convex surface and blunt edges	• Used to separate uveal tissue from sclera during evisceration
Evisceration curette	• Round cup attached to a stout handle	• Used to curette out intraocular contents during evisceration procedure

Table 4.5 (continued)

Instrument	Key features	Uses
Chalazion scoop	• Small cup attached to a narrow handle, smaller than evisceration curette	• Scoop out contents of the Chalazion
Corneal surgery		
Fixation/markers		
Osher-Neumann Corneal Marker	• Marks radial lines on the cornea, semi-sharp blades • Eight lines, inner diameter of blades is 4.5 mm	• Helps in the orientation of sutures and graft during keratoplasty procedures
Hoffer Optic Zone Marker	• Various marker diameters with central crosshairs	• Helps in the orientation of sutures and graft during keratoplasty procedures
Fixation Rings	• Flieringa Fixation Ring available from 15 to 20 mm • Also available with handles that don't require suturing to the sclera	• Helps to secure the globe during open-sky procedures like keratoplasty
Surgical keratometer		
Maloney Keratometer	• A cone-shaped instrument designed to reflect the microscope light in concentric rings on the cornea to detect astigmatism	• Minimize postoperative corneal astigmatism by controlling suture tension during keratoplasty
Miscellaneous keratoplasty instruments		
Teflon block	• Platform made of Teflon	• Used as a base for the donor button before the calibrated punch is used • Always keep donor endothelial side up, minimal touch to the endothelial side during the procedure
Artificial anterior chamber	• It has a mechanism to keep donor cornea in place, while a constant pressure is maintained using balanced salt solution from an infusion line	• Allows dissection on the epithelial side to minimize surgically induced astigmatism • Also allows retrieval of partial thickness grafts
Disposable and suction trephines	• Suction trephines have cutting circular blades assisted by a manual suction mechanism that holds the recipient cornea • Precise cuts with suction trephines ensure uniform, perpendicular cuts • Disposable trephines are used with Teflon blocks for retrieval of donor button	• Trephines help in retrieval of a predetermined circular corneal button for keratoplasty

(continued)

Table 4.5 (continued)

Instrument	Key features	Uses
Glaucoma surgery		
Kelly descemet punch	• Produces round punches without tissue tags • Has serrated squeeze action handles • Two sizes: 0.75 mm, 1 mm punch	• Creation of dural window in optic nerve fenestration surgery • Trabecular meshwork block excision in trabeculectomy
Harms Trabeculotome	• Pointed tips with 3 mm spread; 0.3 mm diameter • Pair consists of right and left	• Sweeping the Schlemm canal in trabeculectomy
Crescent knife	• Single bevel: Crescent bevel up or down angled 45° (20 G) • Double bevel: Crescent bevel up angled 45° (19 G) • For groove or pocket and tunnel incision	• For creating scleral flap or pocket in trabeculectomy and glaucoma drainage device implantation
Tooke's knife	• Short, flat blade with blunt edge	• To separate conjunctiva at limbus during trabeculectomy
Phacoemulsification surgery		
15-degree side port knife	• Straight sharp pointed tip angled 15°	• For side port incisions for introducing irrigation-aspiration handpiece • For doing paracentesis
Keratome Slit Blade	• Disposable; 2.2 or 2.8 mm	• Used for phaco stab incision • Limbal, clear corneal, or near clear corneal incision, which can be biplanar, or three-step incision • Helps to make the incision with lesser force and minimizes wound leakage with minimum SIA
Phaco tip	• Angulation of tip may vary from 0 to 60 deg • More the angulation, lesser the holding power and more the cutting power • Distal opening is the aspiration port • Lateral opening is for irrigation ports • Types of tips: standard tip, Kelman tip, micro tip, micro-flow tip, Mackool tip, ABS tip, Cobra tip, TurboSonics tip • Size of incision depends on tip gauge and sleeve • Hard cataract needs more part of exposed tip, while soft cataract requires less exposed tip	• Acoustic energy produced along ultrasonic handpiece is transmitted onto the nucleus through the tip • Emulsification occurs due to the mechanical jackhammer effect, cavitation bubble, and acoustic fluid wave • Newer tips are offered with additional features like the Stellaris tip (Bausch + Lomb) with power modulation and pulse shaping or Infiniti (Alcon) tip with both longitudinal and torsional (OZiL) ultrasound delivery using a Kelman bent needle and the Whitestar Signature (AMO) tip which has both longitudinal and transversal or elliptical (Ellips) ultrasound delivery

Table 4.5 (continued)

Instrument	Key features	Uses
Wrench	• Device used to remove and fix phaco tips on the handpiece • Is usually handpiece- and manufacturer-specific and employs a screwlike mechanism	• Used during surgery to change tips in case the nucleus is too hard or soft
Phaco sleeve	• Silicon sleeve to cover over the phaco tip • It has two holes on the side, 180 degrees apart • Comes in a wide variety of sizes and colors based on tip configuration • Sizes: 19G, 20G, 21G, and 23G • Autoclaved or ETO sterilized	• Helps to keep the phaco energy localized at the tip • Prevents leakage from corneal wound • Improves nuclear component followbility
Test chamber	• Silicon chamber	• Tuning of the phacoemulsification machine If a small nuclear fragment is stuck in the tip or aspiration tubing, it can be removed with BSS in the chamber, in the energy mode
Osher Y-hook	• Straight arm, blunt two pronged tips • Simple mechanical expansion is done using two Y-hooks	• Used to mechanically dilate the pupil to facilitate more space for the capsulorhexis
Sinskey Lens Manipulating Hook	• Pencillike handle with an angled, blunt, 0.18–0.2 mm tip	• Rotation of nucleus and prolapsing it into anterior chamber • Lens dialing and manipulation
Chopper	• Used for nucleus manipulation procedures like chopping • Named after scientists who invented the technique of use, e.g., Nagahara Chopper, Seibel Chopper, and the Drysdale manipulator	• Used to decrease phaco power as manipulation can help to break down nucleus pieces without phaco power
Mackool-Kuglen hook and IOL rotator	• Angled shaft, rotator tip • Push-pull style	• Used to position IOL and haptics • Retrieve suture from AC
Irrigation/ aspiration handpiece	• Can be bimanual or coaxial • Aspiration is usually 0.75 to 1.5 mm away from tip • Opening can be 0.2,0.3,0.4, or 0.5 mm in diameter • 19G, 21G, 23G, or 25G	• Used to remove cortical matter to facilitate implantation of IOL • Remove excess viscoelastic before end of surgery to decrease inflammation • To polish the posterior capsule
IOL injector	• Plunger or screw style • Slot for insertion of cartridge loaded with foldable IOL • Metallic ones are reusable • Preloaded, disposable are also available	• Used to inject loaded, foldable intraocular lens

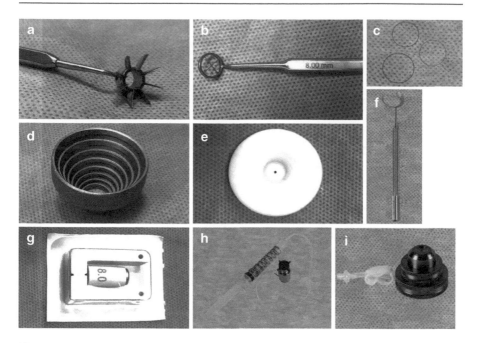

Fig. 4.5 (**a**) Osher-Neumann Corneal Marker; (**b**) Hoffer Optic Zone Marker; (**c**) Fleiringa Fixation Rings; (**d**) Maloney Keratometer; (**e**) Teflon block; (**f**) Fixation Ring with holder; (**g**) disposable trephine; (**h**) suction trephine; (**i**) artificial anterior chamber

Fig. 4.6 (**a**) Steven's Tenotomy Hook; (**b**) Jameson Muscle Hook; (**c**) Chalazion scoop; (**d**) evisceration curette; (**e**) evisceration spatula; (**f**) enucleation spoon

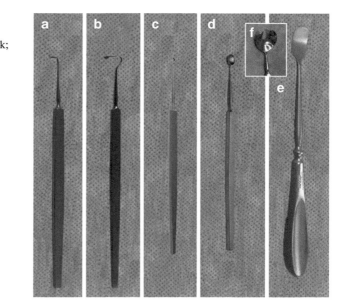

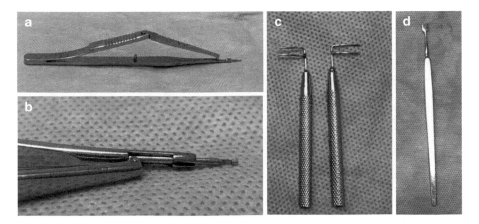

Fig. 4.7 (**a**, **b**) Kelly descemet punch; (**c**) Harms Trabeculotome; (**d**) Tooke's knife

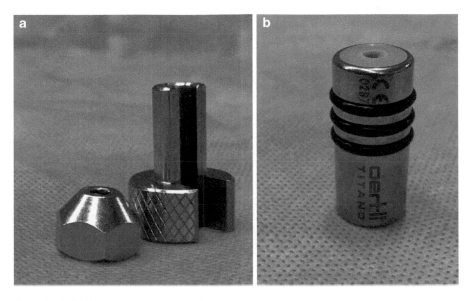

Fig. 4.8 (**a**, **b**) Different types of wrench

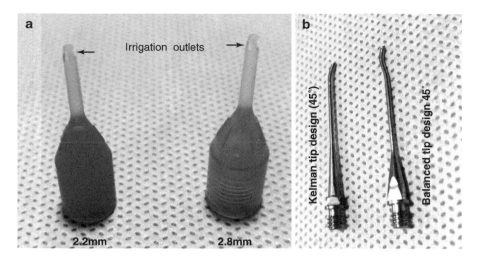

Fig. 4.9 (a) Sleeves; (b) phaco tips

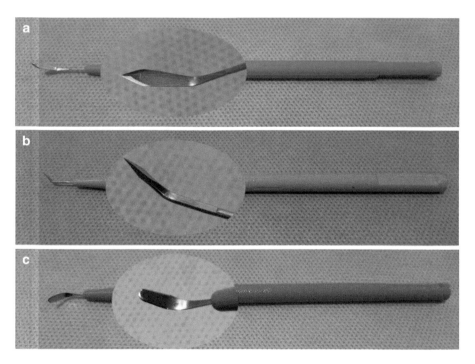

Fig. 4.10 Disposable knives: (a) keratome; (b) 1.5 mm dual bevel side port blade; (c) crescent knife

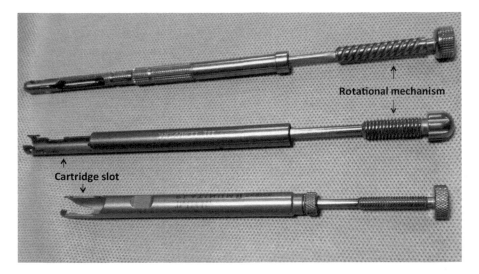

Fig. 4.11   Lens injector systems: rotatory and plunger type

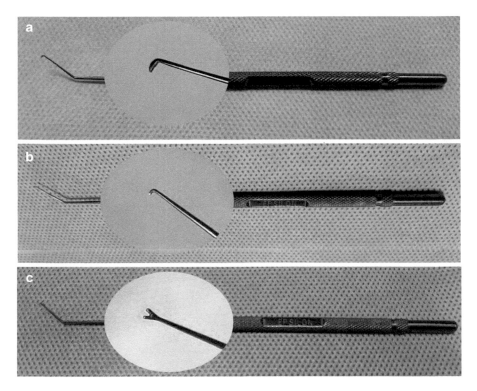

Fig. 4.12   (**a**) Chopper; (**b**) Sinskey hook; (**c**) Osher Y-hook

References

1. Stucky C-CH, Cromwell KD, Voss RK, et al. Surgeon symptoms, strain, and selections: systematic review and meta-analysis of surgical ergonomics. Ann Med Surg (Lond). 2018;27:1–8.
2. Honavar SG. Head up, heels down, posture perfect: ergonomics for an ophthalmologist. Indian J Ophthalmol. 2017;65(8):647–50.
3. Urano T, Kasaoka M, Sagawa K, Yamakawa R. Evaluation of lid speculum with a drape (LiDrape(®)) for preventing surgical-field contamination. Clin Ophthalmol. 2015;9:1227–32.
4. Huang W, Zhang X. 3D printing: print the future of ophthalmology. Invest Ophthalmol Vis Sci. 2014;55(8):5380–1.
5. Gao A, Gonenc B, Guo J, et al. 3-DOF force-sensing micro-forceps for robot-assisted membrane peeling: intrinsic actuation force modeling. Proceedings of the IEEE/RAS-EMBS International Conference on Biomedical Robotics and Biomechatronics 2016. 2016. pp. 489–94.

Instruments for Posterior Segment Surgery

5

Sahil Jain, Mohit Dogra, and Deeksha Katoch

5.1 Introduction

The vitreoretinal surgical armamentarium has undergone tremendous advancement ever since Robert Machemer performed the first vitrectomy using a 17-gauge cutter in 1970. With the advent of the microincision vitrectomy, newer cutter designs, higher cut rates, and better illuminating systems, retinal surgery has undergone a paradigm shift. This chapter aims to provide an overview of the instruments used for posterior segment surgery in today's era.

5.2 Vitreous Cutter

Key Points An instrument with an aspiration tubing attached at one end of the handpiece and extended tube attached to the opposite end of the handpiece. The extended tube has an outer tube and an inner tube. The aspiration tube is attached to vitrectomy machine. These are available in variable gauges (20, 23, 25, or 27 gauge, Figs. 5.1, 5.4) with dimensions of 1.16, 0.75, 0.55, and 0.40 mm, respectively. The distance between the port tip and the cutter opening also varies and shortens as the gauge decreases to allow working closer to the retina.

S. Jain · M. Dogra · D. Katoch (✉)
Department of Ophthalmology, Advanced Eye Centre, Post Graduate Institute of Medical Education and Research (PGIMER), Chandigarh, India

© Springer Nature Singapore Pte Ltd. 2019
P. Ichhpujani, M. Singh (eds.), *Ophthalmic Instruments and Surgical Tools*, Current Practices in Ophthalmology, https://doi.org/10.1007/978-981-13-7673-3_5

51

Fig. 5.1 A 25-gauge
vitreous cutter
(ULTRAVIT,
Constellation, ALCON™)

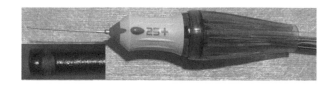

Mode of Working Vitreous is drawn into a port near the distal end of the outer tube. The inner tube moves, occludes the port, and cuts the vitreous. The cut vitreous is then aspirated through the aspiration tubing.

Uses
- To remove the vitreous gel in pars plana vitrectomy for various indications such as:
  - Clearing of vitreous opacities (e.g., hemorrhage, vitritis, degenerations, exudates).
  - In retinal detachment surgery
- As a dissector or an alternative to intraocular forceps in segmentation and delamination of epiretinal membranes in tractional retinal detachments.
- To perform lensectomy
- To make surgical iridectomies
- To perform pupilloplasty
- To perform primary posterior capsulotomy in pediatric cataract surgery
- For surgical capsulotomy

Types of Cutters
- Rotatory: where inner tube spins inside the outer tube and cuts tissue and the port is closer to the tip of probe. They cause more traction on vitreous.
- Guillotine: inner tube moves along a longitudinal axis causing less traction on vitreous.
  - *Pneumatic cutter*: A pneumatic pulse from machine closes the cutter guillotine blade and a spring opens it, but as the cut rate becomes higher, the spring is unable to close the blade resulting in longer time during which port is closed.
  - *Dual pneumatic cutter:* The passive spring return mechanism is replaced by separate air lines to both open and close the vitrectomy port. This allows the duty cycle to be controlled independent of the cut rate with customized modes: "port biased open" or "core" mode (the port remains open for the majority of time), 50/50 mode (the port is open 50% of the time), and "biased closed" or "shave" mode (the port remains closed for the majority of time).
- Hypersonic cutters: These are based on a piezoelectric ultrasound transducer that liquefies the vitreous at the edge of the port. Vitesse hypersonic vitrectomy (Bausch + Lomb) is a prototype of hypersonic cutters. It reaches a much higher cut rate than guillotine-based cutters (up to 1.7 million cuts per minute).

Cut Rate It defines the amount of time port is open. Higher the cut rate, lesser is the time during which port remains open. Thus there is less traction on vitreous with higher cut rates allowing removal of vitreous while working closer to the surface of retina.

5.3   Endoilluminator

Key Points An instrument with a fiber optics attached to one end which connects to the light source in the vitrectomy machine. It provides illumination during vitrectomy. Gholam A. Peyman in 1976 first introduced endoillumination by inserting an optic fiber into the vitreous cavity for a 20-gauge three-port vitrectomy.

Light Sources
The commonly available light sources used for endoillumination are the following:

- *Halogen or metal halide*: This was the most common illuminating source in the 20-g era. With the smaller gauge probes, however, the reduced surface area of the fiber optics resulted in 40–50% less brightness.
- *Xenon*: Xenon light bulbs are the standard illuminating source in the Constellation Vision System (Alcon; Figs. 5.2, 5.4), Stellaris PC (Bausch + Lomb), and Bright Star (DORC, Inc.) vitrectomy platforms.
- *Mercury vapor*: A mercury vapor illuminator (Photon II; Synergetics Inc., St Charles, Missouri) is available which is proposed to provide enhanced illumination with lesser retinal phototoxicity compared to the xenon light source.
- *LED (Light-emitting diode)*: Available on the EVA (DORC, the Netherlands) and the VersaVIT (Synergetics, USA) vitrectomy platforms. LED bulbs offer the advantage of an extremely long life span of more than 10,000 h. These also have built-in filters to minimize phototoxicity.

Types
- Focal illuminators: e.g., handheld light pipes
- Wide angle illuminators: e.g., chandelier illuminators
- Illuminated instruments: e.g., illuminated picks, lasers, scissors, forceps, and infusions

They allow the surgeon to perform bimanual segmentation of membranes and perform peripheral scleral depression in challenging cases.

Uses
- To visualize retinal structures during vitrectomy surgery
- To check the correct placement of infusion cannula prior to the start of vitrectomy

Fig. 5.2 A 25-G endoilluminator (ALCON™)

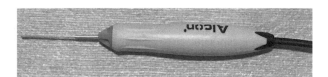

- As a second instrument to provide stabilization in certain cases such as a dropped nucleus in vitreous cavity
- To localize and treat retinal breaks in chandelier assisted scleral buckle surgery
- *Recent Developments*:

   Use of powerful light sources like Xenon and mercury vapor have made microincision vitreous surgery (MIVS) more popular, as they provide the same degree of light in the back of the eye through 25G systems, as was being provided by halogen/metal halide 20G light sources. This has added chandelier endoilluminators to the armamentarium of retinal surgeons. Twenty-five gauge and 27G chandeliers are available, and they allow bimanual surgery in complex cases such as proliferative vitreoretinopathy, giant retinal tears, intraocular foreign bodies, and tractional retinal detachment. Xenon light-based 25G chandeliers provide a cone angle of 79° with a 50% increase in transmission capacity.

Practical Pearls
- Dual 29-gauge chandelier has the advantage of a significantly smaller trochar and diffused light which eliminates the shadowing effect of a single chandelier system.
- Chandelier systems help enhance surgical videos.

Potential Complications
1. *Phototoxicity*: The standard measure of safety of a light source is the aphakic hazard sum. For calculating the safety of a light source, its specific spectral output curve is obtained. The aphakic hazard sum is obtained by the intersection of the spectral curve of the particular light source with the aphakic hazard curve. The aphakic hazard sum can be inversed in order to express the number of lumens that are necessary to create a watt of hazard (lumens/hazard watt). Of more importance to surgeons, however, is the retinal threshold time, which incorporates not just the inherent safety of the light source (aphakic hazard sum) but also the working distance, brightness, cone of illumination used (numerical aperture of the fiber), and the industry standard for toxicity of 25 J/cm^2.

   Light filters are employed to improve the safety of endoillumination and also enhance visualization of specific structures in the posterior segment. Amber, yellow, and green filters are employed by different companies. Amber filter is useful during fluid-air exchange as it reduces glare and also for peeling the internal limiting membrane (ILM) when Brilliant blue green (BBG) dye is used. Yellow filters are said to improve visualization of the vitreous, and green filters are preferred while removing the ILM with most dyes other than BBG.
2. *Retinal tears*: The long fiber-optic tube should always be manipulated very carefully and kept close to the entry port as it can touch retinal surface and cause a retinal tear.
3. *Lens touch*: Manipulating the endoilluminator too anteriorly may inadvertently result in lens touch.

5.4 Trochar/Cannula

Key Points A sharp-tipped trochar along with a cannula mounted over the tip. The hind surface consists of three marks of which two are closely spaced indicating distances of 3.0 and 4.0 mm, respectively. Transconjunctival trochar/cannula systems have reduced the scleral incision diameter reduced from 0.89 mm (20G) to 0.64 mm for 23G, 0.51 mm for 25G, and 0.4 mm for 27G MIVS. These are relatively less traumatic and potentially self-sealing and allow easy interchangeability of instruments and infusion sites improving surgical access.

Valved Cannula System Valved cannulas have small silicone leaflets at the external opening. This modification of the cannula design removes the need for plugs to close the port when not in use. Valves are either cap-like silicone membranes mounted onto the cannulas (Dutch Ophthalmic Research Corporation (DORC), Zuidland, the Netherlands) or built into the cannula head (Fig. 5.3; ALCON) (Figs. 5.4, 5.5).

Advantages of Valved Cannula Systems
- Maintain a closed system, reduce chances of hypotony, and provide stable intraocular pressure (IOP) during the entire surgery.
- Reduce the amount of infusion entering the eye and thereby decrease turbulence.
  High infusion flow can cause direct mechanical trauma to the retina, ballooning of the retina if the infusion is directed toward a retinal break, and turbulence especially when working with perfluorocarbon liquids.
- Reduce the "fountain effect" seen in open cannula systems by preventing egress of fluid during instrument exchange, which can potentially dislodge plugs or cause vitreous or retinal incarceration at the sclerotomy sites.
- Allow surgical maneuvers under silicone oil or PFO that were previously challenging.

Disadvantages
- Valved cannulas can lead to increased friction between the instrument and the valve.
  This is especially true for the soft or flexible tip instruments, such as the soft tip cannula.

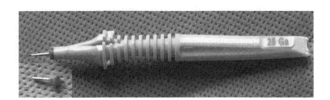

Fig. 5.3 Trocar and cannula system (25g, Constellation, ALCON™). 25G valved cannula in the inset

Fig. 5.4 (From left to right) Assembly of 25-gauge microincision vitreous cutter, endoilluminator, and trocar and cannula system (Constellation, ALCON™)

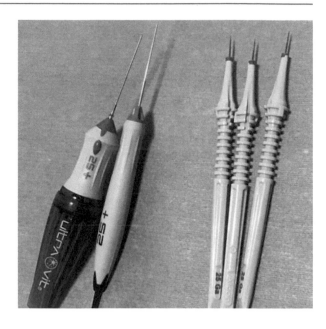

Fig. 5.5 (From left to right) Assembly of 23-gauge microincision endoilluminator, vitreous cutter, and trocar and cannula system (Constellation, ALCON™)

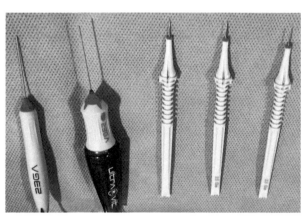

To reduce this a perfectly coaxial insertion approach, augmented with visualization under a microscope, is advocated. Alternatively, displacement of one of the silicone leaflets with a second instrument, such as fine-tipped forceps or use of instruments with shorter, and therefore more rigid, soft-tip extensions and retractable soft tips, is also helpful for insertion.

- Raise intraocular pressure during injection of perfluoro-n-octane (PFO) liquid or silicone oil. Caution is also advised against PFO over fill anterior to the cannula to prevent postoperative retained PFO.

Uses
- To make sclerotomies for microincision vitrectomy surgery (MIVS) procedures
- To mark the distance from limbus for intravitreal injections
- To drain suprachoroidal hemorrhage

Practical Pearl In 20G surgery, the incisions are made with MVR blade parallel to the limbus, while in small gauge (23, 25, 27G) surgery, the trochar incisions are made radial to the limbus.

5.5   Intraocular Forceps

There are a number of intraocular forceps used in microincisional vitreoretinal surgery. Some of the commonly used forceps are listed below.

Key Points It has a handle with different shafts for 20, 23, 25, and 27 Ga surrounded by a stiffening sleeve. The shaft is approximately 27 mm in length. Internal limiting membrane (ILM) forceps have a small, serrated platform at the tip to pinch fine membranes like the ILM (Fig. 5.6). The end grasping and Maxgrip forceps have a stronger hold than the ILM forceps (Fig. 5.7) and are designed to manipulate heavy membranes. They can also be used in various combinations along with the vitreous cutter in bimanual surgery.

Uses
- To peel fine membranes such as:
  - Internal limiting membrane in macular hole surgery
  - Epiretinal membranes
- To hold and remove fibrovascular proliferation (FVP) in cases of diabetic tractional retinal detachments
- To remove lens capsule during pars plana lensectomy
- To pick up dropped intraocular lenses from vitreous cavity
- To use in trans-scleral fixation of IOL
- To peel thick membranes of proliferative vitreoretinopathy

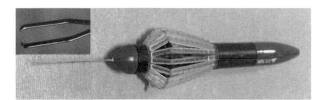

Fig. 5.6 A 27 G internal limiting membrane (ILM) peeling forceps (ALCON, GRIESHABER™)

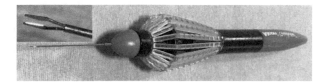

Fig. 5.7 A 25 G end grasping forceps (ALCON, GRIESHABER™)

5.6 Foreign Body Forceps

Key Points A handle with tip mounted on one end and a slider on the body so as to close the tip on to the foreign body surface and hold it. Forceps is available in titanium/stainless steel body (Fig. 5.8).

Use To hold and remove intraocular foreign bodies.

Types
- Claw
- Diamond coated
- Micro-alligator forceps
- Memory snare IOFB extractor
- Quikstik forceps

5.7 Intraocular Magnet

Key Point An intraocular magnet with a steel/titanium shaft. Magnetic tip available in different sizes and a cap to secure magnet to shaft (Fig. 5.9).

Fig. 5.8 Foreign body forceps

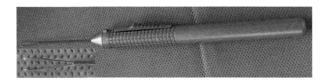

Fig. 5.9 Intraocular magnet

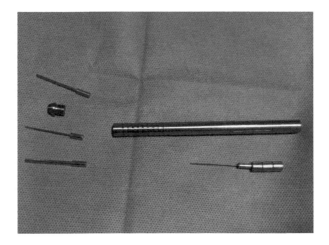

Use To remove magnetic foreign bodies from anterior chamber, lens, vitreous, or retinal surface.

Drawback It cannot be used for nonmagnetic foreign bodies.

Complications
- Retinal tear at site of entry
- Vitreous incarceration of wound
- Trauma to retinal surface (due to inadvertent touch)

5.8   Intraocular Scissors

Key Points The various intraocular scissors available include vertical, horizontal, or curved scissors. Horizontal scissors are angled at 135° with straight blades. In curved scissors there is a curve in the blades to work nearly parallel to the retinal surface and hence reduce chances of impaling the retina with the tips of the scissor. Vertical scissors have angled blades with two fangs. As we press the lever, the two fangs close in anteroposterior direction leading to vertical cut of the structure (Fig. 5.10). These are available in different gauge sizes.

Uses
- Segmentation of fibrovascular membranes in proliferative diabetic retinopathy. In segmentation the membrane is sectioned/cut in-between the epicenters, which are zones of tight adherence often at the blood vessels. Vertical scissor is commonly used for segmentation.
- Delamination: To separate the membrane by shearing from the epicenter. It is used in dissection of thickened proliferative vitreoretinopathy membranes in complex retinal detachments and in proliferative diabetic retinopathy. A curved/horizontal scissors can be used for delamination.

Fig. 5.10 Vertical scissors (ALCON, GRIESHABER™)

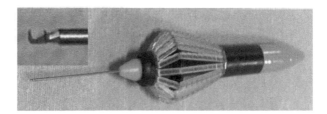

With the recent advances in cutter designs most of the segmentation, delamination is possible with the cutter itself (single instrument) reducing the need for using separate scissors for the purpose except in select cases.

5.9   Miscellaneous

5.9.1   Infusion Cannula

Key Points A 4 mm/6 mm steel bevelled tip fitted at one end of cannula and on other end tip modified to attach to infusion tubing of vitrectomy machine that provides infusion of fluid in vitrectomy (Fig. 5.11). It is imperative to check the placement of the tip of the infusion cannula in the vitreous cavity before switching it on during surgery. Inadvertent placement in the subretinal/suprachoroidal space may result in an iatrogenic retinal/choroidal detachment. Most commonly a 4 mm cannula is used. However in selected situations, a 6 mm cannula may be preferable. These include endophthalmitis where thick exudates preclude visualization and presence of choroidal detachment.

Uses
• To maintain intraocular pressure during vitrectomy
• To infuse air during fluid air exchange
• To inject gas during gas air exchange

5.9.2   Endolaser

Key Point A laser probe with a fiber-optic tip available in 23/25/27 Ga sizes. The tip can be curved or straight (Fig. 5.12).

Fig. 5.11 Self-retaining cannula used in microincision vitrectomy (left), sutured infusion cannula (right), a 6 mm and a 4 mm infusion cannula (inset)

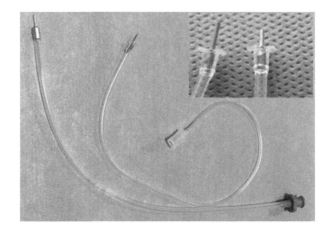

Fig. 5.12 A 25G
endolaser probe with
curved tip (ALCON)

Uses

- To perform intraoperative photocoagulation of retinotomies and retinal tears in retinal detachment
- To perform intraoperative photocoagulation of ischemic retina in cases of proliferative diabetic retinopathy, retinal vascular occlusions, retinal vasculitis, necrotizing retinopathies, and other proliferative vitreoretinopathies

5.9.3 Wide-Angle Viewing Systems

Key Points Wide-angle viewing systems (WAVs) are used for obtaining a panoramic view with easy visualization of the peripheral retina without excessive rotation of the globe during vitreous surgery. Most WAVS consist of two components: an indirect ophthalmoscope lens placed in contact with or above the cornea and a prismatic stereo reinverter that inverts the real image. They can be either contact- or noncontact-type WAVS systems (Fig. 5.13).

- *Contact Lens WAVs*

  Contact WAVS have a fixed field of view depending on the lens dioptric power. They provide better image resolution, contrast, and stereopsis than noncontact systems. This is because they eliminate the natural corneal aberrations and limit the number of reflective surfaces. The main drawback is the requirement of an assistant to hold the lens in complex cases.

  Example: Clarivit and HRX (Volk Optical Inc)

  Various contact lens WAVs along with their specifications are listed in Table 5.1.
- *Noncontact WAVs*

  These do not require an assistant to hold the lens in place. The lens is pre-placed next to the cornea (which gives an inverted image) or a separate prism system to reinvert the image.

  The cornea must be covered by a viscoelastic material or be constantly irrigated to avoid dehydration. Water condensation on the lens is another inconvenience, which requires appropriate draping of the eye. The field of view in noncontact systems varies depending on the distance between the ophthalmoscope lens and the cornea. The field of view may also vary under different surgical conditions: a dilated pupil and an aphakic and air-filled eye may give a wider field of view. Table 5.2 enlists the available noncontact WAVs, while Table 5.3 compares the advantages and disadvantages of contact versus noncontact WAVs.

Fig. 5.13 Noncontact wide angled viewing system (WAVS) RESIGHT 700, Carl Zeiss, Germany with the 128D lens (yellow) and a 60D lens (green). The 128 D lens used for wide angle view and the 60 D lens used for macular surgery

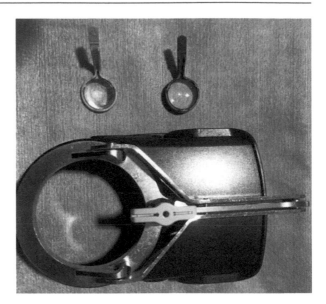

Table 5.1 Contact wide field lenses

Lens name	Manufacturer	Magnification	Field of view (°)
MiniQuad	Volk Optical	0.48×	106–127
MiniQuad XL	Volk Optical	0.39×	112–134
HRX	Volk Optical	0.43×	130–150
Landers WF	Ocular	0.38×	130–146
AVI lens	AVI	0.48×	130–138

AVI advanced visual instruments, *WF* wide field

Table 5.2 Noncontact wide field viewing systems

System	Manufacturer	Maximum field of view (°)
BIOM (HD disposable lens)	Oculus	130
OFFSIS 120 D	Topcon	130
Resight 128 D lens	Carl Zeiss	120
PWL 132 D lens	Ocular	130
EIBOS 2 (132D) Moller-Wedel	Haag-Streit	124

BIOM binocular indirect ophthalmoscopy microscopy, *OFFSIS* optic fiber free intravitreal surgery system, *PWL* Peyman–Wessels–Landers upright vitrectomy lens

5.9.4 Tano Diamond Dusted Membrane Scraper

Key Points This instrument has a soft silicone tip with chemically inert diamond dust at its end. It is available in 20, 23, 25 (Synergetics, Inc), and 27 G sizes (Bausch + Lomb, Katalyst). The metallic dust provides friction and engages the edge of the membrane on the surface of the retina (Fig. 5.14). A retractable version is available to allow easy passage through valved cannula systems.

Table 5.3 Advantages and disadvantages of contact and noncontact WAVs

	Contact lens WAVs	Noncontact WAVs
Advantages	Better axial and lateral resolution, especially at high magnification	Field of view and magnification can be adjusted
	Less need of ocular rotation	Reduced chances of corneal epithelial erosions
	Preferred in highly myopic eyes as they provide better instrument access	No need of a trained assistant to hold the lens in place
		Provide peripheral view of the fundus even in small pupils, air-filled globes, and pediatric patients
Disadvantages	Compromised view in eyes with corneal and lenticular haze/opacity	Learning curve is more than contact WAV
	Chances of corneal deformation and changes in IOP profile	Relatively poor image resolution and depth perception

Fig. 5.14 Tano Diamond Duster Membrane Scraper (DDMS)

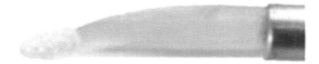

Uses
- Atraumatic removal of ILM and ERM from the surface of retina
- To find the edge of the posterior hyaloid while inducing a posterior vitreous detachment
- To find remnants of the posterior cortical layer of hyaloid adherent to the surface of retina

Practical Pearl
- Long and slow sweeps are preferred over short flicks

5.9.5 Viscous Fluid Injection (VFI) Cannula

Key Points Available in 20, 23, 25, and 27 G sizes for use in MIVS (Fig. 5.15). Allow silicone oil injection and removal through the small gauge cannula systems. They can be directly connected to the silicone oil syringe to allow for manual injection/removal or to an aspiration device connected to the vitrectomy machine.

5.9.6 Gass Retinal Detachment Hook

Key Points A flattened 13 mm Graefe-type hook which possesses a 1.5 mm oval hole at its toe end. Overall length is 5.6 in. and generally has a serrated handle (Fig. 5.16).

Fig. 5.15 (Left to right) 23, 25, 20 G viscous fluid injection (VFI) cannulas

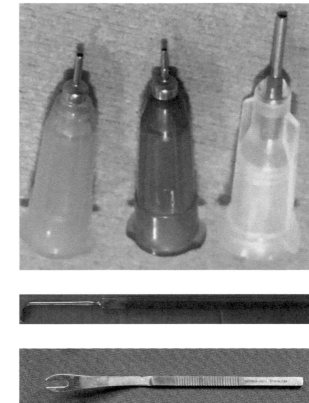

Fig. 5.16 Gass retinal detachment hook

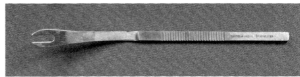

Fig. 5.17 Schepens orbital forked retractor

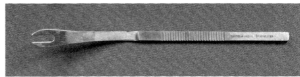

Use
Scleral buckling surgery where a suture can be passed through the hole to allow bridling of the muscles.

5.9.7 Schepens Forked Orbital Retractor

Key Points A retractor with a smooth 14 mm × 56 mm blade having a 4.5 mm wide notch in the blade with a flat serrated handle. Overall length is usually 148 mm (Fig. 5.17).

Use The retractor is especially useful in scleral buckle procedure to retract the conjunctiva and Tenon's fascia to provide adequate exposure of the sclera to pass sutures or tie the scleral buckle.

Suggested Readings

1. Inoue M. Wide-angle viewing system. Dev Ophthalmol. 2014;54:87–91.
2. Mura M, Barca F. 25-Gauge vitrectomy. Dev Ophthalmol. 2014;54:45–53.
3. Osawa S, Oshima Y. 27-Gauge vitrectomy. Dev Ophthalmol. 2014;54:54–62.
4. Shanmugam PM, Ramanjulu R, Mishra KCD, Sagar P. Novel techniques in scleral buckling. Indian J Ophthalmol. 2018;66(7):909–15.

General Instruments for Ophthalmic Plastic Surgeries

6

Manpreet Singh, Manpreet Kaur, Prerana Tahiliani, and Sonam Yangzes

6.1   Introduction

Ophthalmic plastic and reconstructive surgery combines the precision of ophthalmic microsurgery with plastic and reconstructive surgical principles. Basic instruments that form the essential framework of an ophthalmic plastic trolley are discussed in this chapter. Instruments used for oculoplastic surgery are relatively larger and sturdier than instruments for intraocular surgeries but are generally smaller and more delicate than instruments for general plastic surgeries.

M. Singh (✉)
Oculoplastics Services, Department of Ophthalmology, Advanced Eye Centre, Post Graduate Institute of Medical Education and Research (PGIMER), Chandigarh, India

M. Kaur
Glaucoma Service, Department of Ophthalmology, Advanced Eye Centre, Post Graduate Institute of Medical Education and Research (PGIMER), Chandigarh, India

P. Tahiliani
Oculoplastics and Ocular Oncology, Mumbai Eye Plastic Surgery, Mumbai, India

S. Yangzes
Cataract and Refractive Services, Department of Ophthalmology, Advanced Eye Centre, Post Graduate Institute of Medical Education and Research (PGIMER), Chandigarh, India

© Springer Nature Singapore Pte Ltd. 2019
P. Ichhpujani, M. Singh (eds.), *Ophthalmic Instruments and Surgical Tools*,
Current Practices in Ophthalmology,
https://doi.org/10.1007/978-981-13-7673-3_6

6.2   Instrumentation

6.2.1   Bard-Parker Blade Handle

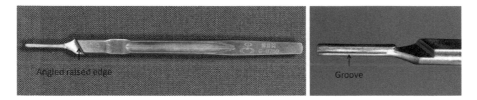

Fig. 6.1   Bard-Parker blade handle

Key Features It is one of the most commonly used surgical instruments which has a flat-serrated or cylindrical-knurled handle for better grip. The business end has a long cylindrical end with two longitudinal grooves on either side for "sliding over" of any scalpel blade. The proximal part has a gap followed by an inclined edge which apposes with the inclination of a scalpel blade (Fig. 6.1). This provides stability to the blade while fashioning an incision. The sterile packing of a disposable plastic handle with a pre-attached blade is also available.

Uses
- Primarily used to mount and handle surgical scalpel blades
- The business end can also be used as guided support while fashioning an incision during the second stage of the Cutler-Beard procedure

Instrument Handling It is one of the first surgical instruments to be handled by budding doctors and all surgeons. The typical pen-holding manner is learned best with it. For the safety of assistants or staff nurses who generally load and remove the scalpel bladed from it, the proximal slant should be matched with that of the BP handle, and the blade is smoothly loaded over the two longitudinal grooves. While removing, a hemostat forceps or a specially designed scalpel blade remover can be used. The pulling out with the hand is strongly discouraged to avoid any injury. The groves should be kept rust free and lubricated.

6.2.2 Foerster Sponge Holding Forceps

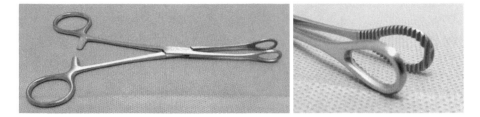

Fig. 6.2 Foerster sponge holding forceps

Key Points This instrument has long blades with oval rim-shaped ends having transverse serrations at both inner surfaces (Fig. 6.2). These serrations provide better grip/hold and the central gap providing sufficient space for sponges to accommodate without draining soaked povidone-iodine solution. The ring handles and ratchet lock system provide sufficient grip to manipulate. This is probably the most commonly used instrument in all surgeries.

Uses
- To clean the target area with povidone-iodine-soaked cotton or gauze piece.
- It can also be used to grasp and hold a large skin flap, atraumatically.

Instrument Handling This instrument is usually safe to handle as its primary use is before starting the surgery. Its other use in ocular surgeries is minimal and could be used for handling large skin grafts. The mucosal handling should be done with care. Ideally, the same sponge holder should not be used for the second patient as this is the first instrument to come in contact with the patient's skin containing microorganisms. Hence, this instrument should not be carried back to the trolley or sterile area and should be handed over for sterilization.

6.2.3   Baby Jones and Backhaus Towel Clamps

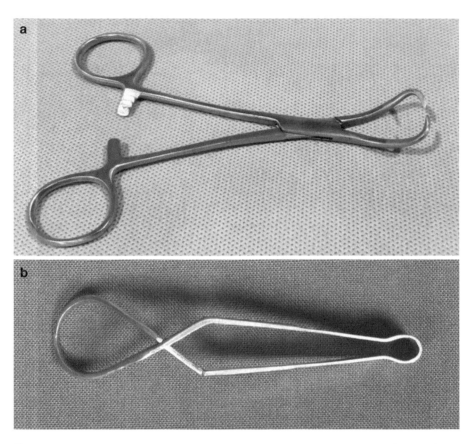

Fig. 6.3 (a) Backhaus towel clamp with ring handles and ratchet locking system. (b) Baby Jones towel clamp with self-retaining system

Key Points Both have sharp, pointed prong tips which overlap for getting locked. The space between the slender curved blades is for accommodating surgical drapes or pipes. The Baby Jones has a self-retaining type of lock mechanism, while the Backhaus has ring handles with ratchet lock system (Fig. 6.3).

Uses
- Used mainly for holding multiple sterilized drapes to prevent intraoperative slippage and exposure
- To hold the wires, cords, suction pipes, phacoemulsification tubings, etc. over the trolley and surgical area for proper handling and care
- The Backhaus clamp can be used to hold/handle skin grafts

Instrument Handling These instruments have sharp, pointed tips; hence these should be used with more caution as it accidentally grips the patient's skin or other tissues while applying over the surgical drapes. This can be a really painful experience for the patients being operated under local anesthesia. To avoid this accidental skin grasp, simply lifting the sheets before locking the jaws may prevent inadvertent injuries. One can also try lifting the drapes after engaging with one of its sharp tips before locking. While enclosing the wires, cords, pipes, or tubings, careful hold under proper visualization is a must to clamp those into the space between two closed blades. A back-and-forth movement of wires ensures its adequate positioning.

6.2.4 Guthrie/Graefe Retractor

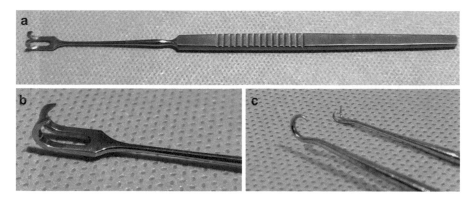

Fig. 6.4 (**a**) Two-pronged Guthrie retractor. (**b**) Close-up of the business-end. (**c**) Graefe single-pronged retractor and Guthrie retractor

Key Features The Guthrie retractor has two small, sharp-tipped, and delicate prongs at its business end with a long holding shaft. The Graefe retractor has a single-hook, sharp-tipped, and stout retractor at its business end with a longer shaft to hold and pull (Fig. 6.4).

Uses
- Mainly used to retract the lower or upper lip during the oral mucosal membrane harvesting procedure for mucous membrane grafting
- To retract small skin wounds for incisional or excisional biopsies
- Can occasionally be used to retract skin or lacrimal sac flaps in external DCR

Instrument Handling After adequate submucosal anesthesia, the retractor tips are applied at the mucocutaneous junction of the target lip. The gentle pull is applied for the retraction of the desired amount to expose sufficient space for harvesting the labial mucosa. Any excessive or jerky force can lead to a mucosal laceration or avulsion injury. The sharp tips provide sufficient strength, and the small prongs leave enough operative space for work. For retracting the skin edges, the tips of the retractor hook should be gently passed over one edge of the incision. Proper care should be taken to avoid any injury to the assistants.

6.2.5 Dieffenbach-Serrafine Bulldog Forceps

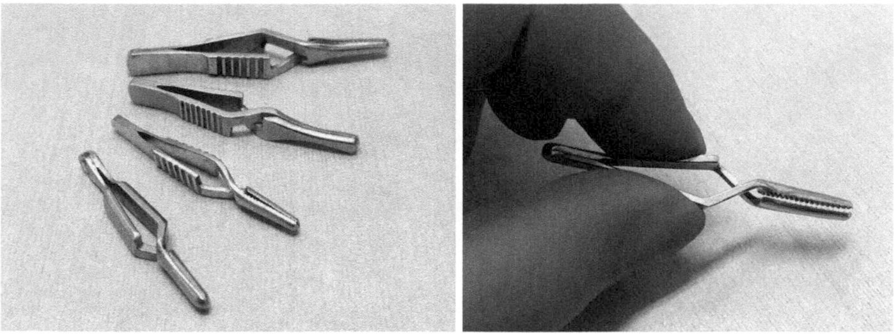

Fig. 6.5 Dieffenbach-Serrafine bulldog forceps

Key Points It is a self-retaining forceps with blunt tips and serrated interlocking jaws (Fig. 6.5). It is one of the smallest surgical instruments on the trolley. To open the jaws, one needs to press the small limbs with fingertips; the jaws close on releasing the pressure. It is available in straight or curved jaws and has an overall length ranging from 38 to 55 mm.

Uses
- To hold and isolate the specific suture threads especially in LPS resection surgery
- Can be used similarly during strabismus, enucleation, and eyelid surgeries
- Can be used to hold the superior rectus traction suture during an ECCE
- Can rarely be used as a small clamp for holding eye drapes, etc.

Instrument Handling Its easy handling, self-retaining nature, and small size make it a user-friendly instrument on the trolley. It is specifically designed to hold the sutures for proper isolation, identification, and manipulation to avoid confusion while handling multiple suture arms in the surgeries mentioned above. The suture arm is always held perpendicular to the serrations for the best possible grip. Once the suture is held in it, the assistant should keep it away from the active surgical field to prevent sudden accidental jerk leading to an avulsion injury. These are very handy and useful in most of the ophthalmic plastic surgeries and constitute indispensable items during some of the mentioned procedures, especially for the beginners.

6.2.6   Bishop Harmon Forceps

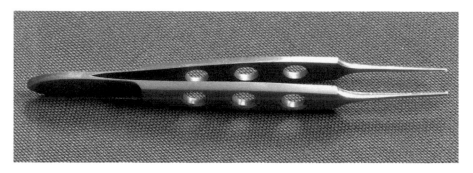

Fig. 6.6 Bishop Harman forceps

Key Points It is a straight-tipped, 2 × 1 toothed forceps with three round fenestrations in both limbs. 0.5 mm from the flat platforms raises the tip (Fig. 6.6). This is one of the most commonly used forceps in ophthalmic plastic surgeries.

Uses
- To hold tissue for a firm grip during intraoperative manipulations
- To reflect the held tissues away or evert it, for a better surgical view
- To hold the eyelids while performing electrolysis, eyelid repair, and various other ophthalmic plastic surgeries
- To hold an orbital mass while an incisional or excisional biopsy
- To hold foreign bodies, tubes, pipes, and drains for various manipulations

Instrument Handling Three circular holes in the limbs make the forceps lighter and provide better grip. It is a toothed forceps; hence the mucosa should not be handled as it may buttonhole or lacerate it. Ideally, the force used to grip any soft tissue should be sufficient only to interlock the teeth of any forceps as any extra force over the limbs may lead to parting/splitting of the teeth. Fragile tissues like cornea and conjunctiva should not be handled with it.

6.2.7   Lester Fixation Forceps

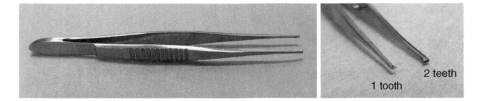

Fig. 6.7   Lester Fixation forceps

Key Points   It is a toothed forceps (1 × 2 teeth) with stout limbs having transverse serrations for better grip of held tissues (Fig. 6.7).

Uses   Similar to Bishop Harmon forceps.

Instrument Handling   Similar to Bishop Harmon forceps.

6.2.8 Graefe Globe Fixation Forceps

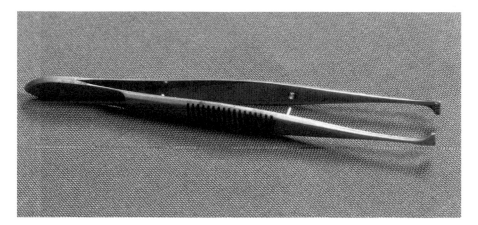

Fig. 6.8 Graefe globe fixation forceps

Key Points It is a stout forceps used to hold delicate tissues in its fine teeth present on the insides of small (3.5 mm) but strong jaws (Fig. 6.8). The limbs or handle has horizontal serrations.

Uses
- To hold the conjunctiva for fixing or holding the globe during any intraocular procedure
- To atraumatically hold the fine skin of eyelids during various surgical procedures
- To catch hold of foreign bodies, stents, tubes, etc.

Instrument Handling It is a recommended instrument to be used for fixing the globe and prevents the torsional or rotatory motions of eyeball during surgical manipulations. The amount of tissue held is greater than a single-toothed forceps, hence better stability. The grasped tissue (conjunctiva or skin) does not get lacerated or torn until gross handling is done. It is not helpful in holding or retracting the deeper tissue along with skin in various ophthalmic plastic surgeries. It is most commonly confused with a multi-toothed forceps which has longer and interlocking teeth and is used for firmer grips of skin and subcutaneous tissue.

6.2.9 Bonaccolto Dressing Forceps

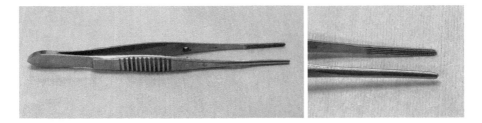

Fig. 6.9 Bonaccolto dressing forceps

Key Points This unique forceps has blunt tips with longitudinal and cross serrations over inner apposing platforms (Fig. 6.9). The limbs or handles have longitudinal serrations for better grip.

Uses
- To hold the lacrimal sac and nasal mucosal flaps while suturing in an external DCR
- It can also be used to hold the periocular skin and LPS aponeurosis during an LPS resection surgery
- It can be used to atraumatically hold the conjunctiva, extraocular muscles, or other soft tissues

Instrument Handling It is held in a pen-holding manner like other forceps, and the same principle of adequate force applies here to achieve the best approximation and tissue hold. Extra pressure leads to opening up or parting of tips. It rarely causes a tissue injury, hence safely used in almost all surgeries. The tissue should be held from the edge for better view and control of movements.

6.2.10 Kelly/Crile/Halstead/Hartman (Mosquito's) Hemostatic Clamps

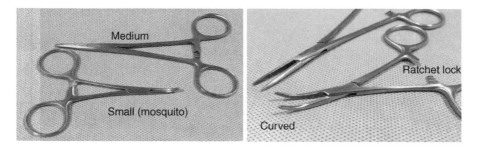

Fig. 6.10 Artery forceps

Key Points These are one of the most sought-after surgical instruments and are considered vital for every trolley due to its multiple uses. Its blunt-tipped jaws have straight or curved shape and are available in small, medium, or large sizes, i.e., from 4.5 to 7.5 cm (Fig. 6.10). These hemostatic clamps have ring handles for better hold and maneuverability, while the ratchet lock system helps to retain the targeted grip.

Uses
Straight jaws:

• To clamp an intact blood vessel, its bleeding end, or a vascular tissue for hemostasis during any surgery
• To crush the lateral canthal tendon during a lateral canthotomy (medium-sized blades)
• To vertically crush the eyelid tarsal plate during eyelid tumor excisions, eyelid reconstructions, etc.
• To crush the extraocular muscles near the insertions during an enucleation or strabismus surgery, for better hemostasis
• Can be used to remove foreign bodies, bone pieces, metal bodkins of lacrimal intubation set, etc.

Curved jaws:

• To hold and crush a bleeding optic nerve stump after enucleation (curved forceps with long blades).
• In Fasanella-Servat surgery for mild ptosis, two small curved artery forceps are used at the superior edge of the everted tarsal plate.
• To hold the orbital fat lobules before excision during a blepharoplasty, orbital fat decompression, etc. to prevent hemorrhage.

Both straight and curved:

- Very commonly used in place of towel clamps, holding the traction sutures with a towel, etc.
- Commonly used to hold small pieces of povidone-iodine-soaked gauze or cotton pieces
- Used to hold a mass, a capsule of a tough-walled cyst, for gentle pulling or manipulations during an excisional biopsy
- Can be used to hold large needles, bend needles of silicone sling, straighten or bend the tip of an instrument, etc.

Instrument Handling   This is one of the most versatile instruments present in a surgeon's armamentarium. The clamping, crushing, holding, dissecting, and gripping effect of its blades are used in desired situations. For the best crushing effect, the tissue should be held twice or thrice with 1–2 mm back-and-forth distance. This consolidates the hemostatic effect of crushing force by clamp's horizontal serrations. A focused suction or hemostasis may provide a sufficient view for adequate time to perform an effective clamping of a bleeding vessel. This end can be clamped with the tip of a straight or curved artery forceps. Now, depending upon the situation, the surgery can be continued, or a cautery can be applied to the base of tissue or the artery clamp itself, for hemostasis.

Multiple artery forceps are needed while performing an orbitotomy or exenteration to hold the tissue/mass, bleeding vessels, and potential bleeders. The holding grip over any tissue, drape, or suture is firm after locking; hence any unwanted jerky/vigorous movement after locking may lead to an avulsion loss of the tissue or suture. The artery forceps can also provide a good blunt dissection effect with its tip. The foreign body, bone pieces, and metal bodkins should be held firmly in the horizontal serrations of an artery forceps for an adequate grip and successful pulling of the material held.

6.2.11 Castroviejo's and Barraquer's Needle Holder

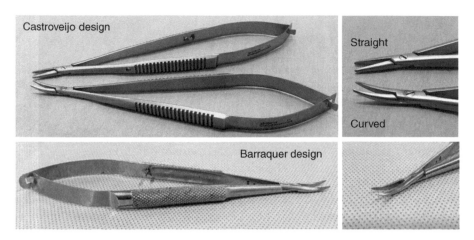

Fig. 6.11 Castroviejo's and Barraquer's needle holder

Key Points The jaws of these needle holders can be either straight or curved but are short, sturdy, and delicate with flat inner platforms. These have spring-leaf type, long handles or limbs. In the Castroviejo type, the handles have transverse serrations, while the Barraquer variant has thick knurled handles; both modifications are for better and controlled grip (Fig. 6.11).

Uses
- To hold the body of a needle for passing it through tissues
- Commonly used to make a needle cystitome of 26 gauge needle tip
- Can be used to hold the suture while tying the knots
- Can also be used to epilate the trichiatic cilia if proper forceps are not available
- Can be used to hold soft tissue like conjunctiva

Instrument Handling   The handles of the needle holder are kept long to provide better hand stability while passing through delicate ocular structures. It also helps in providing desired holding pressure at the jaws with minimum force at handles. The flat inner surface of jaws prevents needle deformation. Generally, the needle should be held at the 2/3rd–1/3rd junction from the needle tip, i.e., at 1/3rd needle length from the swaged end. The spatulated needles have a rectangular cross section which keeps the needle stable and prevents its rotation.

On the contrary, the swaged end and a round-body needle have a circular cross section which can lead to rotation of the needle. Excessive force over the swaged end of a suture can lead to its damage, causing suture loosening, detachment, or breakage. The handles of the needle holder should preferably be without lock while operating under a microscope, to have smooth and non-jerky movements. The needle holders with a lock are generally used by ophthalmic plastic surgeons while operating with a magnifying loupe or the naked eye. Before sterilization, the joint of a needle holder should be properly cleaned for its smooth jaw movements.

6.2.12 Frazier's or Fergusson's Surgical Aspiration Tip

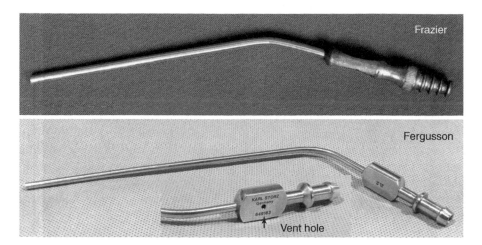

Fig. 6.12 Frazier's and Fergusson's surgical aspiration tip

Key Points It is a long, angled, metallic, hollow suction pipe with a cutoff vent hole over its handle which is controlled with the pulp of thumb. The tip is generally blunt and has 0° angle, and the suction end has metallic corrugations to fit into the rubber hose of the suction pipe (Fig. 6.12). These aspiration tips are available in various sizes for different age groups or depending upon the amount of bleeding. It is popularly called as the "third hand" of the surgeon as it can be used to grasp the soft tissue and pull away for a better view of the deeper tissues.

Uses
- Used to keep the surgical working area clear of blood, blood clots, and debris during routine ophthalmic plastic surgeries (e.g., orbitotomy, orbital exenteration, external and endonasal DCR, etc.)
- Useful in holding the tissues and retrieval of objects lying in the nasal cavity while performing endonasal endoscopic DCR
- Can be used to "vacuum hold" a tissue away (retraction) while performing suction in a deeper region

Instrument Handling This instrument can act as a "third hand" for the ophthalmic plastic surgeon especially while working in deeper spaces. Intraoperatively, it makes the identification of a bleeding vessel easier from a pool of blood and helps in its cauterization. Its tip should be moved cautiously in a blood-filled area as the fragile orbital fat, tissues, and mucosal flaps can get caught and rarely avulsed under high vacuum settings. This happens during an orbitotomy, eyelid surgeries, or DCR. Generally, a medium or low suction pressure is recommended during all ophthalmic plastic surgeries. High vacuum settings can lead to loosening, prolapse, and bleeding from orbital fat while using in orbital surgery. To prevent this, a broad orbital fat retractor facilitates the suction along with good visibility of the operating area.

The most important benefit of suction is that provides a clear field to operate and keeps the surgery proceeding along with the suction of harmful fumes emitted by the cauterized tissue, from the deeper cavities as well as from surroundings.

6.2.13 Castroviejo Calipers

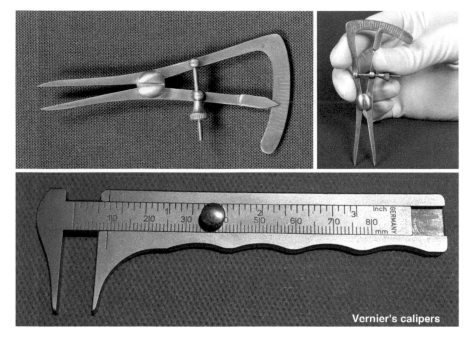

Fig. 6.13 Castroviejo calipers

Key Points It is a measurement device consisting of two limbs, one fixed limb attached to a curved measurement scale usually up to 20 mm (Fig. 6.13). Both limbs have pointed tips for accurate measurement points. Both limbs meet at an angled joint above which an adjustable screw-lock is present to keep the calipers opened at the desired measurement. Usually, the curved scale has markings on both sides, and the pointer on the mobile limb is split to point on both sides of the scale.

Uses
- To measure the size of excised pterygium defect for calculating the graft size
- To measure the amount of extraocular muscle resection or recession in a strabismus surgery
- To measure the dimensions of any eyelid mass or skin lesion
- For intraoperative measurement of the size of a corneal opacity or lesion
- To mark the length of the incision in a scleral incision cataract surgery (for beginners)
- To determine the distance of the site of buckle or band placement in a retinal detachment surgery
- To determine the distance from limbus for intravitreal injections, vitrectomy ports, scleral-fixated lens ports, etc.

- To measure the corneal diameters in children undergoing an evaluation under anesthesia (retinoblastoma, buphthalmos, microcornea, etc.)
- To mark the skin incision site in blepharoptosis surgery
- To mark the amount of muscle or tissue resection in LPS resection and Fasanella-Servat surgeries
- To measure the size of laceration and its distance from the limbus during an open-globe injury repair procedure

Instrument Handling   This is a delicate instrument which is a calibrated measurement device mainly used for intraoperative measurements of various tissues defects and to determine the sizes and measure the distances from anatomical landmarks like limbus and muscle insertions. The tips of this instrument are sharp, and adequate pressure is applied for markings. Surgeons very commonly use a pressure dimple created by its tip as an alternative to the marking ink. Once both tips are at desired marks, the limbs are kept stable, and the reading is quickly noted. Now, the screw-lock is tightened to the target mark, and the calipers are used with ease. Caution—In completely "tips-closed" position, the tip of the pointer should coincide with zero marks on the scale. This ensures proper readings and calibration of the instrument.

6.2.14 Stevens Tenotomy Scissors

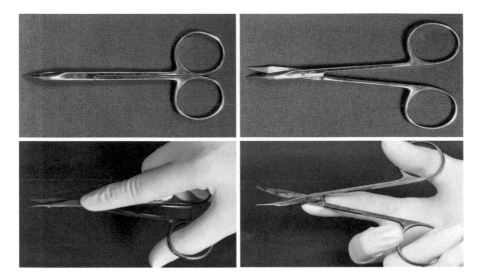

Fig. 6.14 Stevens Tenotomy Scissor

Key Points Tenotomy scissors has blunt-blunt or sharp-sharp tips, stout blades, lap joint and ring handles characterize this instrument. This instrument is one of the essentials in any oculoplastic procedure. The crushing effect of its blades provides sufficient intraoperative hemostasis. The ring handle provides firm grip during the action (Fig. 6.14).

Uses
- To perform the tenotomy (cutting near the scleral insertions) of the extraocular muscles during an enucleation procedure (the instrument is usually named after this procedure)
- To bluntly dissect between the muscle fibers of orbicularis oculi or the orbital septum
- To cut the skin, muscles, and soft tissue during the oculoplastic surgeries
- To create the vertical or horizontal soft tissue planes
- To cut the thicker sutures like 4-0, 3-0 silk or Vicryl sutures
- To undermine the mucosa or skin while harvesting a graft
- To dissect between the sclera and Tenon's during an enucleation or evisceration procedure

Instrument Handling   The blunt-blunt-tipped scissors are preferred for the majority of oculoplastic procedures. The surgeon holds the scissors firmly via the ring handle with one ring occupied by the thumb, and the other can be an index or middle finger as per the surgeon's comfort. The pulp of index finger can be used to support the joint to provide better, stable, and controlled movements for desired outcomes. During an external DCR procedure, after fashioning the skin incision, the closed tip of Stevens tenotomy scissors is placed horizontally through the skin incision, over the bone followed by gentle horizontal separation of the blades to bluntly dissect the orbicularis oculi muscle fibers. This provides sufficient space for the application of the Knapp's cat's paw retractor.

6.3   Practical Pearls

- The instruments should never be passed over the patient's face.
- Blunt tissue dissection minimizes the bleeding—always prefer it over the sharp cutting.
- The blades should be specifically asked only when to be immediately used and should be handed over nurse-to-surgeon and surgeon-to-nurse, with Bard-Parker handle the first position.
- Never use excessive force while using retractors—to avoid tearing the tissues and "caving in" to the undesired planes.
- The needle should be held at a proximal 1/3rd–2/3rd junction in the jaws of the needle holder.
- For hemostasis—adrenaline, thrombin (powder), Surgicel/Gelfoam (before concluding the surgery-clot formation/stabilization), bone wax (for bony bleeds), and fibrin glue can be used.
- A surgeon should be well versed with the principles of tissue handling, wound closure, and reconstructions (flaps or grafts)

6.4   Recent Trends

Adjunctive use of gelatine foam and bone wax helps in controlling the intraoperative bleeding. Bone wax is composed of isopropyl palmitate and beeswax and is useful in controlling the bleeding bone surfaces/emissary vessel openings. Gel foam is a water-insoluble hemostatic agent made from porcine skin and used specifically over or in the soft tissues having potential of bleeding for, e.g., orbital exenteration or orbitotomy. Radiofrequency cautery plays a major role in providing a relatively blood-free field of surgery. In newer agents, microfibrillar collagen, oxidized regenerated cellulose, and oxidized cellulose can be used depending upon the type of surgery.

Suggested Reading

1. Schonauer C, Tessitore E, Barbagallo G, Albanese V, Moraci A. The use of local agents: bone wax, gelatin, collagen, oxidized cellulose. Eur Spine J. 2004;13(Suppl 1):S89–96.

Instruments for Lacrimal Surgeries

7

Manpreet Singh, Varshitha Hemanth, and Prerana Tahiliani

7.1 Introduction

Commonly performed lacrimal surgeries include lacrimal irrigation (syringing), lacrimal and nasolacrimal duct probing, dacryocystorhinostomy (DCR—external and endonasal), dacryocystectomy (DCT), and repair of traumatic canalicular lacerations. This chapter presents a brief overview of the instrumentation involved.

M. Singh (✉)
Department of Ophthalmology, Advanced Eye Centre, Post Graduate Institute of Medical Education and Research (PGIMER), Chandigarh, India

V. Hemanth
Clinical Fellow in Ophthalmic Plastic Surgery, Ocular Oncology and Socket Sciences, L V Prasad Eye Institute (LVPEI), Hyderabad, India

P. Tahiliani
Oculoplastics and Ocular Oncology, Mumbai Eye Plastic Surgery, Mumbai, India

© Springer Nature Singapore Pte Ltd. 2019
P. Ichhpujani, M. Singh (eds.), *Ophthalmic Instruments and Surgical Tools*,
Current Practices in Ophthalmology,
https://doi.org/10.1007/978-981-13-7673-3_7

7.2   Instruments Used in Lacrimal Surgeries

7.2.1   Thudichum Nasal Speculum

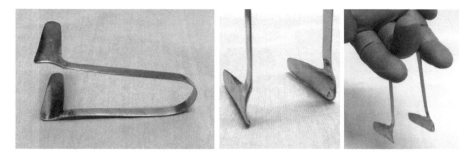

Fig. 7.1 Thudichum nasal speculum

Key Points Its a thin and flexible instrument having two 45–50-mm-long nasal flanges/blades attached to a "U"-shaped handle (Fig. 7.1). The flanges have proximal inner concavities which flatten near the distal ends. It is available in various flange lengths and separates and protects the nasal soft tissues like vestibule, vibrissae, mucosa, etc. from the other operative instruments.

Uses
- Mainly used in OPD for rhinoscopy, nasal foreign body removal, etc.
- Used for facilitating nasal packing before external DCR surgery
- To observe the tip of the lacrimal probe at the floor of the nose in NLD probing
- Can be used to retract orbital fat while removing deep orbital foreign bodies
- To identify and coagulate a bleeding vessel during an orbital surgery
- In short nasal or nasal septum surgeries

Instrument Handling The instrument is generally held in the left hand with its "U"-shaped bent resting over the middle or index finger and is stabilized with the left thumb. The surrounding fingers help in its closure when approximated close to each other. This brings the speculum in its insertion position of closed flanges. After anesthetizing the nasal cavity, the instrument is inserted deep into one side of the nose, and fingers are loosened to open up the flanges. This provides a secured room in the nasal cavity to operate. While taking it out of the nasal cavity, the flanges should be in a semi-closed rather than the closed position to avoid catching hold of any nasal vibrissae or other tissues. Generally, its use is limited for nasal packing and anterior rhinoscopy in an ophthalmic plastic surgery operating room.

7.2.2 Tilley Nasal Packing Forceps

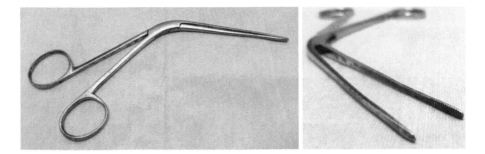

Fig. 7.2 Tilley nasal packing forceps

Key Points It has long and slender limbs with horizontal serrations near the tip, ring handle, and occult lap joint (Fig. 7.2). An angular bent of the limbs provides an unobstructed view of the nasal cavity while manipulating inside; the long and slender limbs help to function in deep and long space like nasal cavity.

Uses
- Used to perform nasal packing with sponge or rolled gauze in DCR surgery
- To remove foreign bodies, crusts, nasal packs, and stents from the nasal cavity
- To remove the bone or cartilage pieces during endonasal DCR and septoplasty
- Can be used to remove deep orbital foreign bodies like wooden, glass, or metallic pieces

Instrument Handling The slender limbs of this instrument should be in a closed position while inserting inside or removing from the nasal cavity. While it is holding any piece of sponge, gauze, mucosa, bone, or cartilage, the blades remain closed. These long blades can also be "opened up" against the medial and lateral nasal walls to provide a transient dilatation to the nasal cavity. While removing the lacrimal stent after 6–8 weeks of nasal intubation, this instrument provides excellent grip to hold the silicone stents for removal from the nasal cavity after the stent loop is cut from the medial canthal region. This instrument can be used with much more versatility for many endonasal endoscopic/non-endoscopic procedures mainly by the ENT and skull base surgeons.

7.2.3 Nettleship/Wilder Single Punctum Dilator/Castroviejo Double-Ended Punctum Dilator

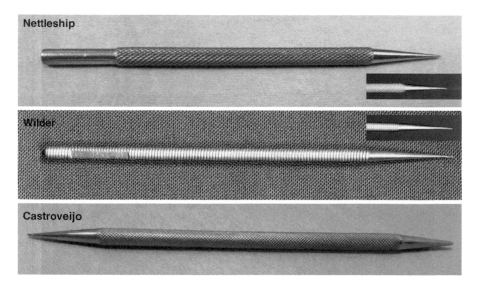

Fig. 7.3 Punctum dilators

Key Points All these dilators are long and slender with tapering pointed tips, available in different sizes of 0.2, 0.3, and 0.4 mm tip diameter, and annular or diamond knurling for facilitating the torsion force leading to rotatory movements during mechanical punctum dilatation process (Fig. 7.3).

Uses
- Diagnostic—before performing any lacrimal irrigation ± probing for the diagnosis of the site of obstruction, it should be mandatory to dilate all the punctum.
- Therapeutic—to mechanically dilate a stenosed punctum as the first line of treatment for mild punctal stenosis.
- To dilate the lacrimal punctum while performing punctoplasty, canaliculoplasty, and nasolacrimal duct probing for congenital nasolacrimal duct obstruction (CNLDO).
- To evacuate or express out the sulfur-granule concretions in canaliculitis.

Instrument Handling Lacrimal punctum dilatation should be performed under proper illumination and adequate magnification (microscope or surgical loupe) for the best outcomes. It avoids an iatrogenic trauma from the tip of a lacrimal probe or cannula which can further cause punctum stenosis or slitting of sphincter/ampulla.

The patient is asked to look in upgaze while handling inferior punctum which is slightly everted with a finger or thumb of left hand. Under topical anesthesia, the tip of punctum dilator is gently inserted perpendicularly into the visible punctal site and rotated to and fro to achieve the desired dilatation. The knurled shaft helps in these gentle rotatory movements. Now, the punctum dilator is tilted horizontally (~90°) along the eyelid margin to dilate the proximal 2–3 mm of the horizontal canaliculus. After removal of punctum dilator, the tip of probe or cannula should be promptly inserted before punctum returns to its normal size. In severe punctum obstruction or atresia, the most probable punctal site (small dimple at the medial end of ciliary row) is tried to open with the sharp tip of punctum dilator or a 26 gauge needle and then dilated in the described manner. The vigorous insertion and rotation are avoided as it can lead to punctum slitting. Serial mechanical dilatations are recommended as first-line treatment for punctal stenosis. Generally, the force required to insert the punctum dilator is provided by its weight; hence no extra force should be applied.

7.2.4   Bowman's or Clarke's Lacrimal Probes

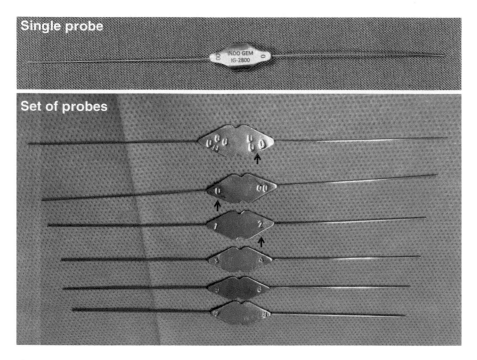

Fig. 7.4 Lacrimal probes

Key Points These are long (~60 mm), sturdy, wire-like, round-tipped probes having two functional sides with a central flat plate for holding it. This plate has markings indicating its diameters (Bowman's—#0000 = 0.7 mm, #000 = 0.8 mm,
#00 = 0.9 mm, #0 = 1, #1 = 1.1 mm diameters) (Clarke's—#00 = 0.6 mm,
#0 = 0.7 mm, #1 = 0.8 mm, #2 = 0.9 mm, #3 = 1 mm diameters). There is a standard
5–10° angulation which is by the direction of the nasolacrimal duct (Fig. 7.4).

Uses
- To perform probing of nasolacrimal duct (NLD) in CNLDO
- To identify and localize the distance of canalicular obstruction
- To diagnose and treat lacrimal canalicular stenosis
- To "tent-up" the medial lacrimal sac mucosa for fashioning lacrimal sac flaps in
  external and endoscopic dacryocystorhinostomy (DCR) surgery
- To do a lacrimal canalicular assessment in cases of canalicular lacerations
- To prevent and identify an inadvertent injury to canaliculus while operating in its
  vicinity (e.g., medial diamond conjunctivoplasty for punctum ectropion)

Instrument Handling After punctum dilatation, the probe is passed smoothly and gently to avoid inadvertent trauma to the canalicular epithelium lining. The anatomical course of the canaliculi should be religiously followed; the first 2 mm is vertical followed by a near perpendicular rotation for its horizontal portion. The probe should lie flat over the eyelid margin, and lateral canthus should be stretched laterally while probing the horizontal canaliculus. This brings the common canaliculus in line with the horizontal canaliculus. On further advancement, a "hard stop" is felt as the probe tip hits the medial wall of the lacrimal sac and underlying bony lacrimal fossa. It obviates any common canalicular obstruction (soft stop).

Probing of NLD in children is usually done through the upper punctum and canaliculus as the lacrimal sac and NLD is more in continuation with superior canaliculus allowing a more accessible entry and rotation of probe. It also safeguards the inferior punctum and canaliculus from any iatrogenic trauma, as inferior canaliculus provides significant tear drainage. After reaching the "hard stop," the probe is withdrawn for a millimeter and rotated superiorly to lie vertically at the superior orbital notch. Now, the probe gently pushed inferiorly into the NLD following its direction (lateral and posterior). The membranous obstructions are felt, noted, and overcome with minimal force. The false passage should be avoided at each step by being adequately gentle and nasal endoscopic guidance. Serial dilatation with larger diameter probes is also recommended in patients with CNLDO.

7.2.5 Modified Worst's Pigtail Lacrimal Probe with Eyelet

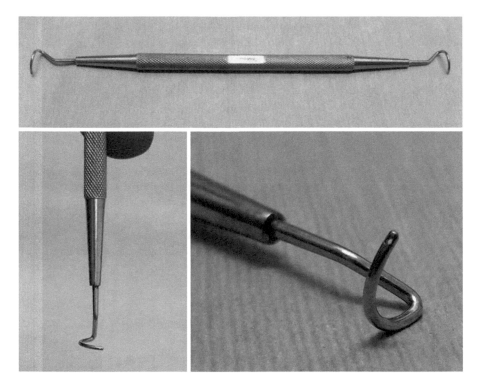

Fig. 7.5 Pigtail probe

Key Points This instrument has a long knurled shaft having pigtail-shaped probes at two business ends; the pigtail probes have a round atraumatic tip, round/oval eyelet near the tip (Fig. 7.5). One needs to identify the side of the probe to be used before its insertion. One business end can be used for superior punctum/canaliculus of one side (right side) and inferior canaliculus of the other (left side) and vice versa. A gentle, rotatory motion is desired.

Uses
- Mainly used in lacrimal canalicular lacerations to identify the lacerated medial end where the direct and indirect methods for localization have failed
- To pass a silicone stent or nylon suture in a railroad method from the lacerated punctum/canaliculus and through the intact opposite punctum/canaliculus

Instrument Handling Note: An intact opposite punctum and canaliculus is necessary to use this instrument. The opposite intact punctum is dilated; some viscoelastic is injected to lubricate the canaliculus. Then, the tip of the pigtail probe is gently inserted and advanced in a smooth rotatory motion without any undue force or stretch to prevent false passage. Eventually, the tip of the pigtail probe should come out from the occult medial end of the opposite lacerated canaliculus. The procedure should occur without much resistance. Gentle, soft tissue tug is felt when the bend of common canaliculus is being traversed. Anatomically, the presence of a common canaliculus is the basic requirement of the procedure to succeed. To-and-fro movements are helpful for successful guidance and outcomes. Once it comes out of the desired location, the suture or a taper-cut stent is threaded via its eyelet, and the probe is reverse passed and taken out from the intact punctum/canaliculus. The use of a pigtail probe is not advised by many, but it may act as a saving instrument in the situation where all other methods to localize the medial lacerated canaliculus fails.

7.2.6   Freer's Double-Ended Periosteum Elevator

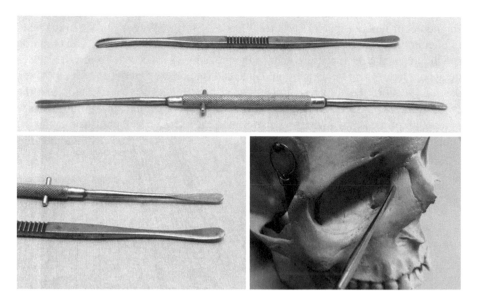

Fig. 7.6 Freer's double-ended periosteum elevator

Key Points It is a long, stout instrument with double end that gives more versatility of using sharp or blunt tips, and the shaft is serrated or knurled for better grip (Fig. 7.6). The sharp tip can act as a cutting tool and avoids shredding of the periosteal edge. The two small horizontal protrusions point towards the sharper tip end. The blunt tip provides atraumatic lift and dissection, and an extra bent can be used as a "seeker" to dissect between maxillary-lacrimal sutures in endoscopic DCR.

Uses
- Used to elevate the periosteum off the maxillary bone in DCR surgery.
- It can be used to reflect the lacrimal sac laterally along with periosteum from lacrimal sac fossa.
- It can be used to create the first opening through the bony suture of lacrimal sac fossa.
- To lift periosteum in orbital exenteration and orbital wall fracture repairs.
- To lift the nasal mucoperiosteum during endonasal DCR.
- It can be used to do blunt dissection around the soft tissue masses/tumors while doing excisional biopsy or orbitotomy.
- It can be used as a blunt soft tissue retractor in small incision surgeries.

Instrument Handling The instrument should be held firmly in a pen-holding manner at the middle knurled or serrated shaft. In external DCR, after fashioning an incision over the periosteum with a no. 15 blade or the sharp edge of the elevator, the periosteum is lifted by the firm and small movements of the blunt-edged end of the elevator. The periosteum is gently scraped off from the bone and reflected to prevent its injury and loss during bony ostium formation. While lifting the periosteum, one must ensure the integrity of its edge as shredding is one of the complications causing improper wound closure. In endonasal DCR, the sharp tip is used to reflect the muco-periosteum, and the extra bent of the blunt end is used as the suture seeker and opener. The blunt tip can be used to flatten the opened up lacrimal sac flaps and appose them with the nasal mucosal edges.

7.2.7   Knapp's or Rollet "Cat's Paw" Retractor

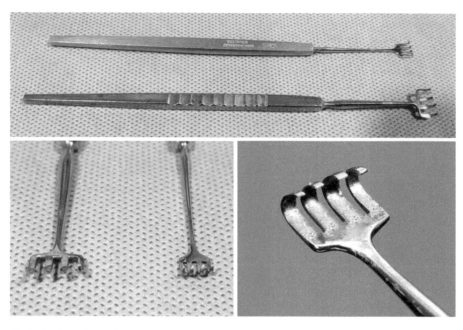

Fig. 7.7   Knapp's "cat's paw" retractor

Key Points   It is a blunt-tipped, claw-shaped, soft tissue retractor with 3-4-5 prongs. It is available in small, medium, and large sizes (used according to the incision size) (Fig. 7.7). It keeps the skin, muscle, and periosteum retracted away from the actual surgical field, and it has a flat serrated handle for a firm grip.

Uses
- To retract the skin, muscle, and periosteum in external DCR procedure
- To retract soft tissue in an orbitotomy, routine ophthalmic plastic surgery procedure
- To retract the tough contracted scar tissue in case of skin grafting
- To temporarily compress a bleeder vessel in the soft tissue during a DCR
- To retract and lift the soft tissue simultaneously, during any surgery (firm grip)
- To retract skin and muscle while harvesting fascia lata from thigh region for frontalis sling surgery

Instrument Handling   While used in an external DCR surgery, the retractor should be applied to the skin, muscle, and periosteum. Its retracting force should be adequate while using single or two retractors, and excessive force may lead to ragged skin wound extension, edge avulsions, and injuries at wound edges. The accidental holding of lacrimal sac mucosa or nasal mucosa into the prongs can lead to the mucosal laceration or mucosal flap avulsion. Accidental slippage while applying excessive force for retraction may cause surrounding soft tissue or eyeball injuries. Intermittent relaxation in sync with the surgeon provides relaxation to the tissues and the assistant's arm. Generally, two retractors are required for each wound edge during any surgery. Both retractors shall work in tandem to facilitate the surgeon by providing the view of the desired site.

7.2.8 Kerrison's/Citelli's Bone Rongeur or Punch/Bone Rongeur

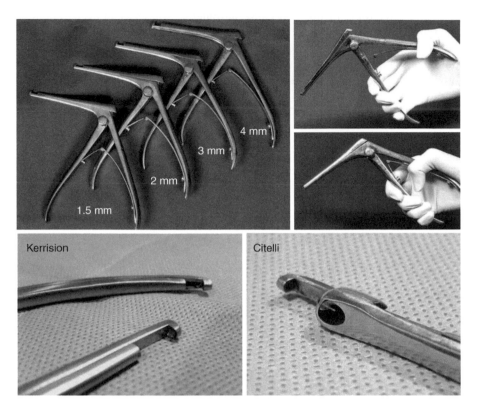

Fig. 7.8 Kerrison's/Citelli's bone rongeur or punch/bone rongeur

Key Points It is a sturdy instrument with two handles (grooved/plain, with/without a horn) and a double spring with the ball-and-socket or pronged joint (Fig. 7.8). The diameter of its tips ranges from 1.5 to 4 mm and is used according to the size of the bony ostium. The rongeur is used for external DCR while with longer limbs is used in endonasal DCR. The upper limb is shorter and sliding, and its tip has an inverted "U"-shaped sharp cutting edge. The lower arm is more extended and fixed, and the tip has a fixed, stout, elevated end with a small cup-shaped depression to accommodate the punched bone piece. For endonasal procedures, the arms are long and slightly curved for better access at a remote area in a narrow nasal cavity. Downcutting and rotatory rongeurs are also available.

Uses
- Used to create and enlarge a bony ostium in cases of dacryocystorhinostomy (DCR).
- It can be used to punch out the irregular bone in old displaced orbital fractures.

- It can be used to enlarge the bony opening to remove the muscle from floor fracture, frontal bone reduction in orbital decompression, etc.
- Used to punch the overhanging orbital rim for better access to the lateral/superior tumors and during the initiation of keyhole osteotomy.
- It can be used to take a biopsy in bone tumors.

Instrument Handling This instrument should be held most firmly as it needs a considerable amount of force to punch the bone (easier in children and difficult in adults). At the beginning of the bony ostium, its tip should be introduced gently through a small bony opening made with a bone awl or Freer's periosteum elevator through the innominate suture between maxillary and lacrimal bone. The smallest rongeur (1.5 mm) goes first and makes the opening large enough for bigger rongeurs. While going through the bony ostium, one should take care not to pierce through the nasal mucosa which lies abutting the bone. Inadvertent injury can happen which can be predicted with the sudden onset of significant bleeding in a previous "dry" area. The tip of the instrument is blunt with round and smooth surface and helps to push the intact nasal mucosa away while it is being inserted. The space between two blades is used to engage the edge of the bony ostium and then close it safely. One should take care not to involve the innocuous nasal mucosa along with the bone. This prevents the concealed enlargement of mucosal defect beneath the bone. A rare event of nasal septal injury or perforation might be encountered on rough usage.

The cutting action is of more importance as it prevents the extra, ragged, and unplanned bony removal which if happens near the skull base can lead to inadvertent dura mater injury and CSF leak. Hence, the rongeur should be closed entirely to ensure a proper "cut" than a break of the bone.

7.2.9 Kilner's Double-End Retractor

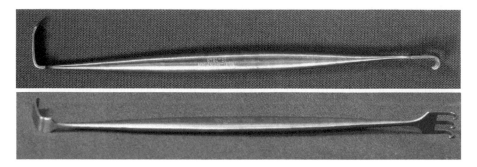

Fig. 7.9 Kilner's double-end retractor

Key Points It is a double-ended instrument, a cat's paw or claw-shaped hook retractor at one end and a long "L"-shaped perpendicular retractor at the other (Fig. 7.9). The long retractor has an inward bend at its tip for better containment and grip of the held soft tissues.

Uses
- To retract the skin, muscle, and periosteum in a DCR surgery (like Knapp's lacrimal sac retractor).
- The "L"-shaped longer retractor side is helpful for deeper tissue retraction (e.g., orbitotomy, orbital floor repair, etc.).
- To harvest the fascia lata for frontalis sling surgery.

Instrument Handling The claw-shaped end has sharper and longer retractors as compared to Knapp's lacrimal sac retractors, and proper care should be observed while handling it. When the claw is in use, the L-shaped end provides a better, longer, and comfortable grip to the assistant for holding the instrument without slippage. However, while using the L-shaped end for retraction, the claw-shaped end should be handled with care as it may cause potential injury to the assistant's hands. This inadvertent injury can be prevented by properly wrapping a cotton gauge piece around the claw retractor end before use. It is a useful instrument in many ophthalmic plastic surgeries including DCR and orbitotomy.

7.2.10 Howard's Bone File

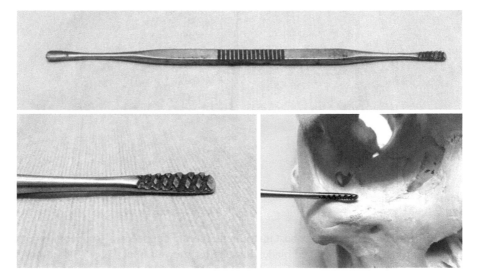

Fig. 7.10 Howard's bone file

Key Points It is a double-ended, long, and stout instrument and has blunt edges to prevent soft tissue or mucosal injury, and one face of the flat end has deep crisscross serrations to file the bony irregularities (Fig. 7.10).

Uses
- To smoothen the bony osteotomy margins in external DCR
- To file the sharp edges of old healed orbital bone fracture or after osteoma removal
- To retract soft tissues in any orbitotomy procedure
- To bluntly dissect out a smooth and firm orbital mass (serrations provide better grip during manipulation)

Instrument Handling The major role of this instrument is to file the sharp traumatic edges of a bone. It is held firmly from the serrated shaft and is moved to and fro at the sharp edge of the bone in a filing motion to smoothen the possibly traumatic edges. According to various studies, the smooth edges of bony osteotomy promote the healing by primary intention and avoid a mucosal laceration. Though the tips have blunt edges, any rough movement/handling can inadvertently cause surrounding soft tissue injury reminding us about the desired short to-and-fro movements. Moreover, the crisscross serrations may be helpful in dissecting and "rolling out" a solid mass from the orbital cavity.

7.2.11 Friedman Bone Nibbler

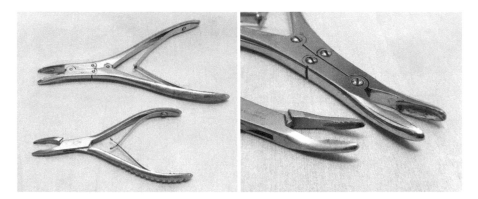

Fig. 7.11 Friedman bone nibbler

Key Points It is a stout and robust instrument, having cupped oval-shaped tips with sharp cutting edges and curved blades for a better view of bone (Fig. 7.11). It has a double-spring action handle and can have box lock or double action joints for handling more amount of force.

Uses
- To nibble the sharp pointed ends of the vertical bones (maxillary process) in DCR procedure
- To remove a part of orbital bone infiltrated by carcinoma
- To take a biopsy from the bony orbital lesion
- To punch out any bone which is thick for Kerrison's lacrimal bone rongeur

Instrument Handling The handles of the instrument should be held firmly, and the pressure is applied in a homogenous way to nibble-cut the projecting bone. This linear force distribution leads to the cutting action of the edges of oval cups, rather than the chipping and breaking of bone pieces. The aim is to smoothly chop off the sharp bone edge from the underlying main bone without disturbing its other bony suture attachments. It is particularly helpful in DCR surgery for removing the vertical and thicker portion of maxillary bone, which does not get engaged into the Kerrison's bone rongeur.

7.2.12 West's Lacrimal Bone Gauge, Chisel, and Mallet (Hammer)

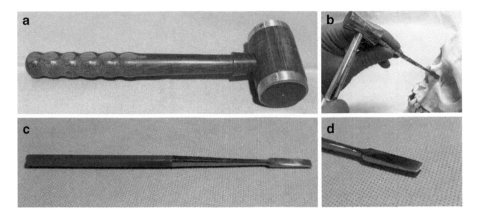

Fig. 7.12 (**a**) Wooden mallet. (**b**) Metallic hammer and chisel in action replica. (**c**) Bone chisel. (**d**) Tapered business end of the chisel

Key Points Chisel is a long and stout instrument with ~20 × 6 mm single-bevel blade at the business end. The beveled edge is sharp and straight to produce a linear impact on the target bone. Mallet is just like a hammer made up of steel and has a heavy bi-headed business end and a thick knurled handle for good grip (Fig. 7.12).

Uses
- To start a bony ostium in DCR surgery while encountering a very thick bone
- To enlarge the bony ostium in case of a very thick maxillary bone
- To handle the bone tumors (osteomas)
- To shape or cut the bony prominence in case of an orbitotomy or decompression

Instrument Handling These instruments are the most sturdy and most massive to be handled by an ophthalmologist. Therefore, these should be held firmly and used carefully as it can injure the surrounding delicate soft tissues with slightest of defocused impact. Though used mostly as a last resort to tackle a tough and thick bone while performing DCR, their function is unique. The patient under local anesthesia should be informed about the instruments feel and sound produced on its use. The gauge or chisel is placed firmly over a marked bony area. The area of the target should preferably be rough, and a guide mark can be carved onto the bone with chisel edge to prevent its slippage. This is a good exercise for better control in the small working area. The mallet is held in another hand, and the initial impact should be with minimal force. This is to avoid a catastrophic unexpected bony, mucosal, and nasal septum perforation.

7.2.13 Shahinian's/Bailey's Lacrimal Irrigating Cannulas

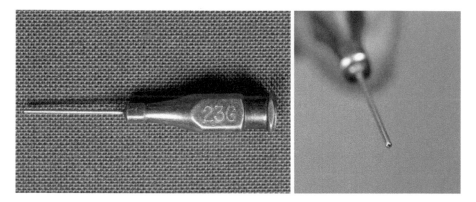

Fig. 7.13 Lacrimal irrigating cannulas

Key Points The lacrimal irrigating cannulas have smooth, tapered edges which are gentle and atraumatic to the epithelium lining of lacrimal canaliculus. Shahinian—11 mm (tapered end); Bailey—7 mm (bottlenecked end), 23-gauge diameter each (Fig. 7.13).

Uses
- To perform lacrimal irrigation for the diagnosis of the lacrimal obstructions
- To ensure the anatomical patency of the mucosal communication between the lacrimal sac and nasal cavity after DCR procedure
- To confirm the opening of a canalicular obstruction after performing a canalicular trephination
- To confirm the patency of a nasolacrimal duct with fluorescein dye in a child after performing probing (not an essential step though)

Instrument Handling The cannulas should be well polished with smooth finishing to avoid any mechanical trauma to the canalicular epithelium lining. Ideally, the cannula should be straight with a tapered end. This facilitates the directional movement of the cannula, and minimal resistance of the canaliculus is encountered. While performing lacrimal irrigation, the patient should be preferably in a supine position. Punctum dilatation with a punctum is a norm. The lacrimal cannula mounted on a 2 cm^3 syringe filled with normal saline should be gently introduced and proceed. Mild force should be used to inject the fluid while performing intra-canalicular or intra-sac irrigation. The patient subjectively confirms for the passage of fluid into the nasopharynx. Both puncta should be observed for the regurgitation of fluid in canalicular or nasolacrimal duct obstructions.

7.2.14 Stevenson's/Agricola's/Muller's Self-Retaining Lacrimal Sac Retractors

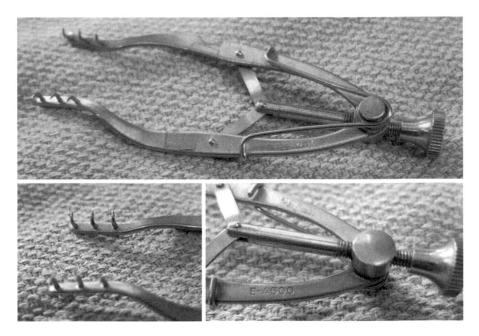

Fig. 7.14 Stevenson's self-retaining lacrimal sac retractor

Key Points The self-retaining feature keeps the hands of surgeon and assistant free for rest of maneuvers. The tips of prongs are blunted to avoid soft tissue damage, spring base (Agricola) and screw base (Stevenson) joint (Fig. 7.14). The limbs of Agricola retractor have two semicircular plates for pressing the limbs. A length of 20 mm and 32 mm tissue retraction is provided by the Stevenson and Agricola tissue retractors, respectively.

Uses
• To retract the skin and muscle in external DCR especially with an untrained assistant
• To retract the soft tissue in dermoid cyst excision surgery
• To retract the skin and muscle in incisional biopsy of orbital masses

Instrument Handling These retractors are less commonly used by the ophthalmic plastic surgeons as the flexibility of operating field view is compromised during the extra-dynamic surgery like DCR. Self-retaining lacrimal sac retractors need to be applied in a closed limb position into the wound edges. This is done by pressing the limbs between thumb and index finger (Agricola) or unscrewing Stevenson's limbs, before insertion. The hold and tissue application should be firm and stable to prevent the accidental slippage or dislodgment causing an injury to the surrounding soft tissue or eyeball. The joint between two limbs should be kept either toward forehead or inferiorly to avoid field obstruction. Overall, the use of Stevenson's retractor is more controlled than other retractors. The need for assistance is reduced in external DCR or short duration surgeries, and the assistant is free for suction or other routine assistance.

7.2.15 Arruga's Lacrimal Trephine

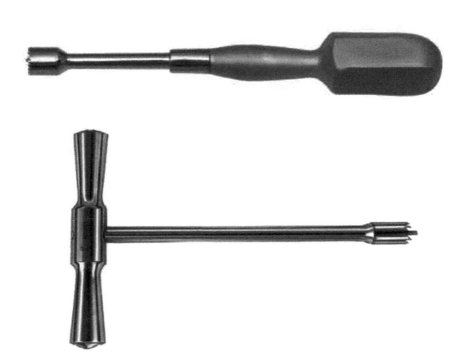

Fig. 7.15 Arruga's lacrimal trephine (Image Source: Ovation International; Microtrack Surgicals)

Key Points This is a historical instrument having a "T" shape or straight shaft. The business end had a hollow cylindrical flare with its edge having deep and sharp serrations (Fig. 7.15). A sharp central pin acted to pierce and grip the trephined bone segment. The diameter ranged from 7 to 10 mm.

Uses
• To punch out a bony ostium of the desired size in primary DCR surgery.
• To enlarge the pre-existing bony ostium in secondary DCR surgeries.
• It was rarely used to take a punch biopsy from a bony lesion.

Instrument Handling The instrument with a central pin was used for primary DCR surgeries in which the bone used to be intact, while the "without-pin" model would have been useful for enlarging the previous DCR bony ostium. The "T"-shaped handle would have been helpful in providing the necessary rotatory action. A mild medially directed force would have helped to punch out a circular bony opening. An excessive force could lead to sudden perforation of bone and injury to the nasal mucosa or inadvertent perforation of nasal septum. Due to this potential dreaded complication, nowadays, its use is minimal, and this instrument is mostly of historical value.

7.2.16 Recent Trends

Use of monocanalicular or bicanalicular stents during punctum, canalicular, lacrimal sac, and nasolacrimal duct related procedures is a common adjunctive addition. Use of the nasal endoscopic system is on the increase among the oculoplastic surgeons which helps in the management of these disorders in a minimally invasive manner. The details about the nasal endovision system are mentioned in another chapter. Use of adjunctive agents like mitomycin-C has been considered to provide better success in dacryocystorhinostomy.

Suggested Reading

1. Singh M, Kamal S, Sowmya V. Lacrimal stents and intubation systems: an insight. Delhi J Ophthalmol. 2015;26(1):14–9.

Nasal Endoscopic System

8

Manpreet Singh and Saurabh Kamal

8.1   Introduction

The nasal endovision system or the nasal endoscopy unit is a useful addition to the oculoplastic clinic due to its prominent role in the disorders of the lacrimal sac and nasolacrimal duct. Its role in the preoperative evaluation of the nasal cavity before primary or revision, endonasal or external DCR, postoperative ostium evaluation, and monitoring of the lacrimal stents, is of paramount importance. Moreover, its role in the management of failed probing or persistent congenital naso-lacrimal duct obstruction (CNLDO) has been established to look for and manage the inferior turbinate or inferior meatus-related factors responsible for the failure of previous probing(s).

The operating surgeon (right-handed) always stands on the right side and vice versa for the left-handed surgeon. The endoscope is held in the non-dominant hand, and the other instruments for intranasal manipulations are handled by the dominant hand.

Potential uses of the nasal endovision system in ophthalmology:

- Endoscopic endonasal DCR (primary or revision)
- Endoscopy-guided lacrimal intubation or balloon catheter dilatation for persistent CNLDO
- Endoscopic orbital decompression for thyroid-associated orbitopathy
- Endoscopic optic canal and optic nerve decompression
- Harvesting the nasal mucosa or septal cartilage for grafting
- Obtaining a specimen for the suspected cases of mucormycosis
- Postoperative examination for the DCR ostium (endo or external)

M. Singh (✉)
Oculoplastics Services, Department of Ophthalmology, Advanced Eye Centre, Post Graduate Institute of Medical Education and Research (PGIMER), Chandigarh, India

S. Kamal
Ophthalmic Plastic Surgeon, Eyehub, Faridabad, Haryana, India

© Springer Nature Singapore Pte Ltd. 2019   113
P. Ichhpujani, M. Singh (eds.), *Ophthalmic Instruments and Surgical Tools*,
Current Practices in Ophthalmology,
https://doi.org/10.1007/978-981-13-7673-3_8

8.2   Basic Nasal Endovision System

8.2.1   Hopkins II Rigid Telescope

This is the business end of a functioning nasal endovision system. The length of this medical-grade, stainless steel telescope rod ranges from 175 to 180 mm (Fig. 8.1a). It consists of a metallic, rigid pipe attached proximally to an eyepiece lens (Fig. 8.1a, black portion). Near the eyepiece, a perpendicular attachment is present for the connection of the fiber-optic light pipe to the telescope (Fig. 8.1b). The eyepiece has a sapphire lens to provide excellent image quality. The metallic pipe contains a "rod-lens system" which focuses the image at the eyepiece, which gets conveyed via the camera to the monitor.

The tip of the telescope has a central (0°) or eccentric (30°, 70°) lens (Fig. 8.1c) for viewing, surrounded by the illuminating micro light tips (Fig. 8.1d) which are ends of the optical fiber bundles. The tip has an antireflective coating protecting this sensitive structure from the mechanical micro-abrasions which can have a permanent impact on the image quality. The telescopes are available in two diameters for the endonasal procedures—2.7 and 4 mm Fig. 8.1c. The variable angulations of the tip (0°, 30°, 45°, and 70° Fig. 8.1d) are available in both 2.7 and 4 mm telescopes. Zero-degree scope provides the "end-on" view, while 30-, 45-, and 70-degree scopes provide the respective "angled" view. A colored ring is used at the base of the light pipe attachment post—green for 0°, red for 30°, black for 45°, and yellow for 70° telescopes.

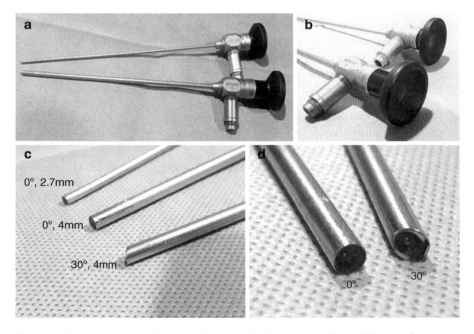

Fig. 8.1 Hopkins II rigid telescopes. (**a**) Two rigid telescopes (above-2.7mm, below-4mm), green- 0 degree and red- 30 degrees. (**b**) The eyepieces showing the quartz lenses in the center. (**c**) Various types of telescopes. (**d**) The ends showing the arrangement of lenses at the tips of 0 and 30 degree telescopes

Routinely, the 2.7 mm scopes are used for diagnostic endoscopy/diagnostic rhinoscopy—for preoperative assessment, postoperative evaluation, stent removal, and nasal endoscopic guided probing/intubation/balloon catheter dilatation for CNLDO. The 4 mm scopes (more rigid and sturdy than 2.7 mm) are used for routine endonasal endoscopic DCR, laser DCR, conjunctivo-dacryocystorhinostomy with tube placement, etc.

It was used to be kept in a formalin chamber and saline cleaned before use. Nowadays, plasma sterilization and the autoclaving option are available for few of the company products. Fogging over the telescope viewing end occurs during diagnostic rhinoscopy and surgical procedures. It is caused by an imbalance between the temperature of the front lens, the temperature of the nasal cavity, and the humidity of the environment. It results in condensation of moisture over front lens of a telescope. Also, blood, debris, and mucosal secretions can further stick and get dried over the lens, disturbing the view. Commonly, the chlorhexidine and cetrimide solution (marketed as Savlon by GlaxoSmithKline limited), baby shampoo, or povidone-iodine can be used as antifogging agents for cleaning the tips. Antifogging is a crucial step to get the best possible image quality for better outcomes, especially in the early stages.

8.2.2   Fiber-Optic Light Pipe

This delicate and compact bundle of special optical fibers transmits the halogen or xenon light from the source to the endoscope, for illumination of the nasal cavity. The outer material is made up of silicone, polyvinyl chloride (PVC) (Fig. 8.2), or flexible metal; first two materials are preferred to avoid any electric short circuit

Fig. 8.2 Fiber-optic light pipe

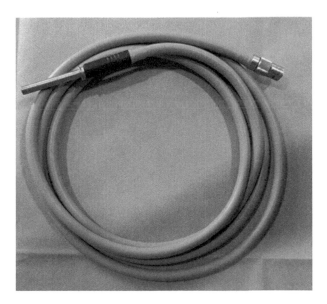

chance. The wavelength of the light transmitted ranges from 380 to 1500 nm—xenon in "pulse" and halogen in "continuous" form. Fused fiber end of the light pipe can withstand the temperature up to 250 °C. Routinely, 4 mm diameter light pipe is sufficient for nasal endoscopic surgeries like DCR, FESS, septoplasty, etc. This delicate wire does not withstand any undue mechanical abuse like stretching, pulling, acute kink, or puncture, which might result in irreversible damage to the optical fibers. The xenon light source bulb stands approximately 30,000 h with 300 W of power.

Of the two ends, the longer, metallic, rod-shaped end goes into the light source unit, while the other smaller end (with grooves) is attached to the Hopkins II telescope with a screw lock adapter.

8.2.3   Camera Head

Modern compact design and modified camera heads provide more extensive uses to the surgeon. A charged-coupled device (CCD) camera with single-chip (Fig. 8.3a), 3-chip, or full-HD (1920×1080 pixels) recording system is available which mounts the eyepiece of the Hopkins II telescope. The camera head forms the major bulk which is held firmly by the operating surgeon (with non-dominant hand) during the endoscopic surgery. It has got a white balance button, recording button, and zoom button over its anterior surface (Fig. 8.3b, c).

Near its attachment for the telescope, the camera head has one rotating dial for focusing and another dial for zooming (in case of a single-chip camera, Fig. 8.3c). Camera and telescope should be attached and rotated to get the correct position and

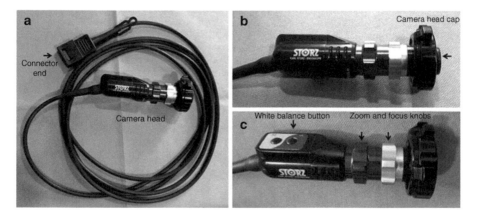

Fig. 8.3 (a) Camera head with wire and connector end. (b) Side-view of the camera head with cap to protect the front lens. (c) Top-view shows the buttons and knobs

orientation ensured by upside-down and sideways movements. The Image 1-S technology® is provided by the Karl Storz® for HD recording of surgical procedures in a 2-D or 3-D format. It has got an inbuilt parafocal zoom lens (up to 5×) with a focal length of 15–31 mm.

8.2.4 Cold Light Fountain Unit (Fig. 8.4)

Three types of light sources are available, halogen, xenon, and LED. The halogen provides good quality of light at 3600°K temperature and 250 W power, while xenon lamps burn at 5600°K and provide pure light for better color distinguishing. The LED is the latest (6400 K) and most efficient form of a light source having least maintenance, economical, and environment-friendly. These days the portable LED light sources are also available like our routinely used power banks for mobile phone charging. These portable LED light sources when fully charged provide the light with 100% intensity for 90–120 min.

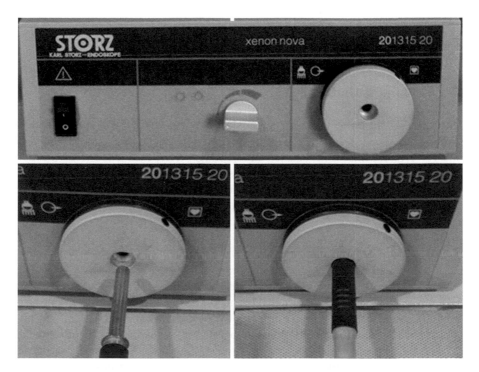

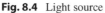

Fig. 8.4 Light source

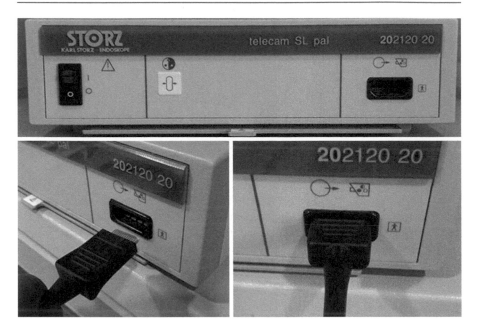

Fig. 8.5 Camera unit

8.2.5   Camera Unit

The camera unit has got an attachment slot at the front for the connector end of camera handpiece. The front surface of this unit may have a digital or analog module for controls like white balance and shifting the type of video (NTSC/PAL). Figure 8.5 demonstrates the orientation, insertion, and final position of the connector end. The camera and cold light source units should be kept well-aerated for adequate temperature maintenance and interference-free operation.

8.2.6   Display Monitor (Fig. 8.6)

The medical-grade, 2-D or 3-D monitors with wide-field viewing (16:9 aspect ratio) are best to provide a view from an HD camera head and Hopkins II telescope rod-lens system. High color contrast provides the best details about the blood vessels, and the vital structures present inside the cavities especially in a blood-stained field.

The final attachment of the camera head, optical light pipe, and telescope is shown in Fig. 8.7 the crucial joint where the surgeon holds the endoscope during all the procedures, ergonomically. The telescope is an optically and physically delicate item which should be dealt with utmost care. The white balancing should be done whenever the camera unit is switched on. Figure 8.8 shows the assembled nasal endoscopic system and a procedure underway.

Fig. 8.6 Display monitor with recorder, camera unit, and light source

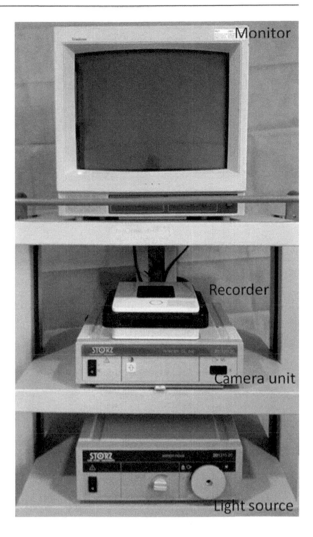

Fig. 8.7 Joint where the surgeon holds the endoscope during all the procedures

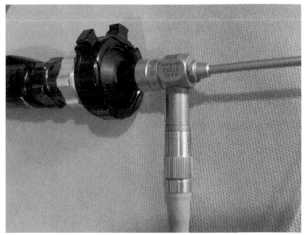

Fig. 8.8 Nasal endoscopic
procedure underway

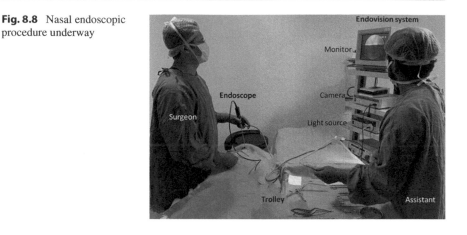

Suggested Reading

1. Ali MJ. Nasal endoscopic setup. In: Ali MJ, editor. Atlas of lacrimal drainage disorders. Singapore: Springer; 2018. p. 49–60. https://doi.org/10.1007/978-981-10-5616-1_4.
2. Curragh DS, Halliday L, Selva D. Endonasal approach to orbital pathology. Ophthalmic Plast Reconstr Surg. 2018;34(5):422–7.
3. Saleh H, Choudhury N. Setup for nasal endoscopy and endoscopic surgery. In: Ali MJ, editor. Principles and practice of lacrimal surgery. Singapore: Springer; 2018. p. 75–80.

Instruments Used in Eyelid Surgeries

9

Manpreet Singh, Varshitha Hemanth, and Prerana Tahiliani

9.1   Introduction

Blepharoptosis correction, surgeries for entropion or ectropion, chalazion incision and curettage, eyelid mass excision and reconstruction, blepharoplasty, and epilation are commonly performed eyelid surgeries.

Characteristically, the skin of the eyelid and the periocular region is thin and loose which makes it difficult to fashion a smooth and superficial incision over it. Hence, the skin is held stretched between index finger and thumb of the non-dominant hand, and the base may be supported by a sturdy, smooth, and flat instrument. For exact localization, the skin should be marked with a fine-tipped surgical skin marker, without stretching and before local infiltration anesthesia. This avoids erroneously longer or shorter eyelid incisions leading to inappropriate results.

M. Singh (✉)
Oculoplastics Services, Department of Ophthalmology, Advanced Eye Centre, Post Graduate Institute of Medical Education and Research (PGIMER), Chandigarh, India

V. Hemanth
Clinical Fellow in Ophthalmic Plastic Surgery, Ocular Oncology and Socket Sciences, L V Prasad Eye Institute (LVPEI), Hyderabad, India

P. Tahiliani
Oculoplastics and Ocular Oncology, Mumbai Eye Plastic Surgery, Mumbai, India

© Springer Nature Singapore Pte Ltd. 2019
P. Ichhpujani, M. Singh (eds.), *Ophthalmic Instruments and Surgical Tools*,
Current Practices in Ophthalmology,
https://doi.org/10.1007/978-981-13-7673-3_9

121

9.2   Instrumentation

9.2.1   Snellen Entropion Clamp

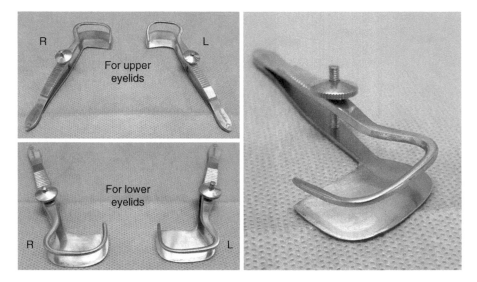

Fig. 9.1   Snellen entropion clamp

Key Points   It has a "U"-shaped superior rim and a "D"-shaped inferior plate as a continuation of upper and lower handles, respectively. The plate provides a flat base and acts as a globe protector, while the rim acts as a hemostasis clamp. The portion inside the rim is the field of work. It has a screw mechanism to tighten both limbs after its correct application, and the handle is always kept temporally. So, one clamp can be either used for upper eyelid of one side and lower eyelid of the contralateral side (identification is important).

Uses
- To provide adequate globe protection and eyelid hold during eyelid surgeries specially entropion/ectropion corrections
- To provide intraoperative hemostasis during eyelid surgeries
- Acts as a helpful tool while operating over eyelids without a skilled assistant

Instrument Handling   To determine the side of this instrument, the "D"-shaped plate and "U"-shaped rim are always kept toward the globe and eyelid skin, respectively. The open end of "U" determines the operating area. The handle is always kept toward the temporal side. Hence, the clamp for right upper eyelid can also be used for left lower eyelid surgery, and it is not possible to use it for left upper or right lower eyelid surgery (Fig. 9.1). The cornea should always be anesthetized, and preferably a viscoelastic material or ointment should be applied at the lower base of the plate to prevent an accidental corneal abrasion. The tightening of "U"-shaped rim compresses the peripheral arcade of blood vessels leading to intraoperative hemostasis. It is wise to loosen the clamp before putting closing sutures to locate and cauterize any active bleeding vessels. The removal of the clamp should be smooth and gentle to prevent any corneal or wound injury. Intraoperative contact with the radiofrequency cautery tip or excessive heat can be harmful to the corneal surface.

9.2.2   Jaeger/Berke-Jaeger/Khan-Jaeger Eyelid Plate

Fig. 9.2 Jaeger eyelid
plate

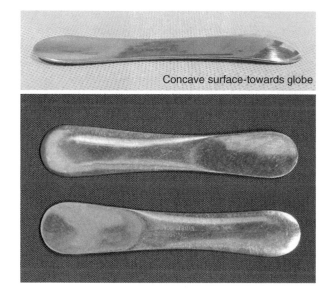

Concave surface-towards globe

Key Points It is a flattened, double-ended, ~100-mm-long platelike instrument with
two different sized blade widths at both ends – for pediatric and adult eyelids. It is a
universal instrument which can be used for either side or eyelid. It has two surfaces, a
convex and a concave, the latter comes in contact with the cornea (Fig. 9.2). Its convex
surface should be dull or sandblasted to minimize intraoperative light reflections.

Uses
- To provide stability while fashioning an incision over the eyelid skin
- Provides stability and supports to the tarsal plate while incising it partial or full
  thickness
- Protects the eyeball from the sharp needle of silicone rod/Wright's ptosis needle
  while making a pass from eyelid to eyebrow or vice versa
- Can also be used as a fat retractor during an orbitotomy
- Can be used as a platform for debulking/cutting skin or mucous membrane grafts

Instrument Handling The ocular surface should be adequately anesthetized, and
the patient should be informed before inserting the plate beneath the eyelid. A
lubricating ointment or viscoelastic gel is applied over the concave surface of the
plate which comes in direct contact with the cornea. The convex surface faces the
eyelid and provides a proper contour and support for surgical maneuvers. The
assistant holds the other end in a spoon-holding manner between the thumb and
index finger (fulcrum). Minimum force is applied to lift the eyelid/tarsal plate to
make it taut and bring it away from the ocular surface. The accidental touch of
radiofrequency cautery tip or excessive heat can be passed onto cornea in a deleterious manner. Hence, the maneuver mentioned above is vital during such activities.
Sandblasting or tilting negates the intraoperative light reflections.

9.2.3   Stallard Ptosis Plate

Fig. 9.3 Stallard ptosis
plate

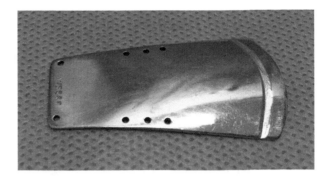

Key Points This is a universal instrument. It is a small plate with a curved and straight end; the curved end has a crescent-shaped groove, while three holes are present on each side in the middle part of the plate (Fig. 9.3). On both sides of the straight end, one hole each is present. The superior or anterior convex surface is sandblasted for reducing the light reflections.

Uses
- To provide stability and support while fashioning incisions over the eyelid skin and tarsal plate
- Protects the eyeball from sharp ptosis needle or blade tips
- Can be used as a platform for cutting skin grafts

Instrument Handling The necessary handling steps remain same as for the Jaeger eyelid plate. The holes are provided to pass the threads of traction sutures applied to the eyelid margin. This helps in keeping the eyelid stretched as well as prevents the sutures from coming in the surgical field and getting accidentally severed. It provides lesser difficulty to the inexperienced assistant while assisting during a dexterous eyelid procedure.

9.2.4   Beer/Barraquer Cilia Forceps

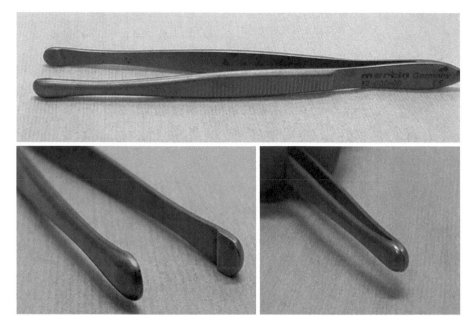

Fig. 9.4   Beer cilia forceps

Key Points   These forceps have short and stout handles with a round to oval-shaped tips (Fig. 9.4). Both inner surfaces have flat platforms for firm grip or hold of an eyelash base. The Barraquer cilia forceps has long, tapered, and angulated tips to provide a better view of the trichiatic eyelashes.

Uses
- To perform manual epilation in patients with trichiasis/distichiasis.
- To remove the eyelashes during electrolysis procedure.
- It can also be used as an adjunct to handle sutures while tying or removing.

Instrument Handling   This forceps is held in a pencil-holding manner in the dominant hand. The eyelid margin is gently everted with the finger of another hand, and the trichiatic lashes are localized under magnification. Now, the forceps are used to hold the abnormally directed eyelash at its base. The base of cilia is at the eyelid margin from where the maximum amount of force can be transmitted to the root of an eyelash and, hence, achieves desired results of complete epilation of the cilia. The tips of eyelashes are thinner and fragile, which should not be held as it can lead to an incomplete removal and breakage of cilia. This leads to the formation of a sharp edge of broken eyelash which rubs in a more deleterious manner over the corneal epithelium than a normal eyelash. It should be inspected in the closed position under magnification to detect any gap or incomplete apposition of platforms.

9.2.5 Lambert/Desmarres/Hunt/Cauer Chalazion Forceps

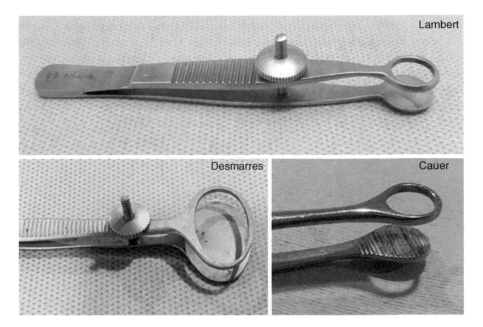

Fig. 9.5 Lambert, Desmarres, and Cauer chalazion clamps

Key Points This is a universal forceps having a same diameter plate and ring at the ends of each limb. The screw lock provides the grip/hold of the tissue. The configuration of plate depends on the surgeon's preference with no significant advantage of one over other (Lambert (round), Desmarres (oval), Hunt (angulated limbs), and Cauer (serrated inner surface of the plate) (Fig. 9.5)).

Uses
- Used in incision and curettage of the chalazion
- Can be used to perform canaliculotomy and curettage
- Can be used to excise small or localized eyelid masses
- Can be used to ensure hemostasis while performing an incisional or excisional biopsy of an inflamed or vascular eyelid mass

Instrument Handling The location of chalazion over the eyelid skin should be marked with a surgical marker pen before infiltrating the local anesthesia. This helps in the localization of the area of interest. With both limbs open and keeping the ring toward the conjunctival side, the clamp is applied. The plate always faces the skin during incision and drainage of chalazion. After instillation of topical anesthesia, the ring is inserted beneath the eyelid guided by the externally marked chalazion site. After ensuring adequate centralization, the screw is slowly tightened, and the eyelid is everted sufficiently to provide an adequate blanch. Now, the tip of surgical blade no. 11 is used to give an incision at the point of maximum height or visible pus point. The incision should be fashioned parallel to the direction of surrounding meibomian glands. This orientation avoids the inadvertent injury to surrounding meibomian glands, creates a less irritant vertical scar, and opens up the gland in the whole length. The spontaneous extrusion of the cheesy material from the incision site provides sufficient evidence of the target. Now, the pressure drainage and curettage is completed. The everted eyelid is moved back to normal position, and the screw is loosened and clamp removed in a quick but gentle movement. Pressure is applied over the eyelid to minimize and stop bleeding.

9.2.6 Meyerhoefer Chalazion Curette

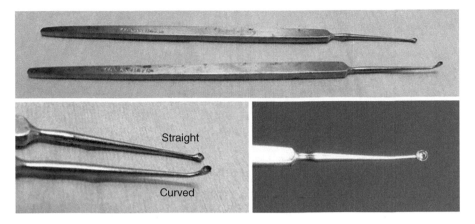

Fig. 9.6 Meyerhoefer chalazion curette

Key Points This is a delicate instrument with a long shaft and a small curette at the tip of its business end (Fig. 9.6). The edges of the round cup-shaped curette are generally sharp, and it may be available in various diameters (1–3.5 mm). The Skeele curette has typical serrated edges which might prove traumatic to the surrounding tissues of tarsal plate, hence less commonly used.

Uses
- To curette out the lipo-granulomatous material from chalazion.
- To remove any impacted foreign body over the tarsal plate.
- Larger (3.5 mm) curette can be used to remove residual focal uveal tissue during an evisceration.

Instrument Handling After giving an incision over the chalazion, the chalazion curette is inserted into the cavity of the blocked meibomian gland. Then the curette is moved all around inside the cavity to break all micro-septae or loculi. This ensures proper evacuation of the contents and prevents the recurrence or residual chalazion at the same site. The lipo-granulomatous material from the curette cup can be sent for histopathology in selected cases like recurrent or multiple chalazia, elderly patient, etc. The tip should be adequately cleaned and protected from mechanical trauma for best surgical outcomes.

9.2.7 Desmarres Eyelid Retractor

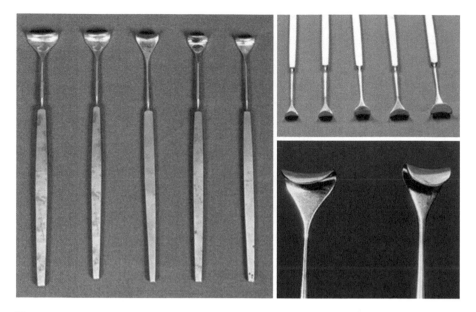

Fig. 9.7 Desmarres eyelid retractor

Key Features This retractor has solid, thin, smooth "C"-shaped blades with blunt edges. The horizontal width of blade decides the retractor size, i.e., size 0 = 11-mm-wide, size 1 = 13-mm-wide, size 2 = 15-mm-wide, and size 3 = 17-mm-wide blade (Fig. 9.7). The concavity at the front end of retractor provides space for inspection and surgical manipulations while keeping the tissues retracted atraumatically.

Uses
- To perform retraction of the eyelid skin, muscles, and superficial fat while performing eyelid or superficial orbital surgeries
- To open single or both eyelids of an uncooperative patient for basic ocular evaluation (eyelid or facial burns, spasm due to foreign body, etc.)
- To perform "double eyelid eversion" for detecting any foreign body in superior fornix/washing of chemical deposits in ocular chemical injuries
- Can be used to insert or remove an ocular prosthesis or contact lens in uncooperative patients
- To perform eyelid retraction of both eyelids during short surgical procedures
- For ocular inspection of a patient with severe blepharospasm

Instrument Handling *For eyelid retraction*: After ocular topical anesthesia, the edge of Desmarres retractor is gently inserted over the upper eyelid margin and is slowly retracted toward the superior bony orbital rim. This opens up the palpebral fissure, and now the second retractor (preferably smaller) is inserted for the lower eyelid. The direction of movement for both retractors should be aimed to lift the eyelid away from the globe slightly. This ensures better exposure, view, and safety. For a quick but magnified examination, the light source and magnifying loupe of hand-held slit lamp should be kept ready. This needs good cooperation from the patient.

For double eversion of the eyelid: The patient keeps the eyelids closed and is continuously directed to relax as forceful closure will not allow a proper examination. The Desmarres retractor is held in a vertical position over the closed upper eyelid keeping its edge near the superior border of the upper tarsal plate. Now, the eyelashes are held, and the eyelid is everted over the retractor. Keeping it in position, now the handle of the instrument is lowered over the eyebrow and forehead. This exposes the superior fornix and conjunctiva allowing removal of any lodged foreign body or accumulated chemical debris.

9.2.8   Berke's Ptosis Clamp

Fig. 9.8 Berke's ptosis clamp

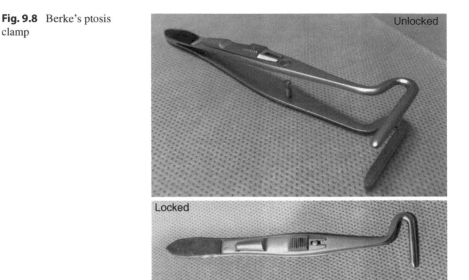

Key Points This clamp has two "L"-shaped blades with transverse serrations on inner surfaces. The upper limb has a slide lock and hole, while the lower limb has a small vertical pillar to accommodate the lock (Fig. 9.8). The blades' lengths range from 20 to 27 mm and are selected according to the patient's age. The tip of blades points nasally, hence for the right and left upper eyelids; two different clamps should be used, as the slide lock should be kept superiorly.

Uses
- To hold the LPS aponeurosis for better anterior and posterior dissection/manipulation during LPS resection surgery.
- It can be used for isolating LPS from other tissues during an anterior orbitotomy.
- Can be used in LPS resection, LPS advancement, and LPS disinsertion repair surgeries.
- Rarely, can be used to hold a rectus muscle while operating over or around it.

Instrument Handling After the adequate exposure of LPS aponeurosis, two full-thickness openings are made at the nasal and temporal ends/horns of levator aponeurosis just above the superior tarsal border. Now, a plane is dissected between the LPS and conjunctiva-Muller's muscle with Westcott's scissors. Before completely taking out the blades of scissors, the inferior limb of the clamp is passed from the temporal toward the nasal opening. This passage should be gentle and smooth without any extra force to prevent a false passage or conjunctival perforation. The handles are always kept temporally for better maneuverability and surgical exposure. Once the end of the clamp is passed beneath the aponeurosis, both limbs are joined, and the slider over the handle is pushed forward to lock the handles. The transverse serrations prevent accidental slippage of the LPS aponeurosis. Once correctly held, the LPS aponeurosis is incised free from the tarsal plate, followed by anterior and posterior dissections from the orbital septum and Muller's muscle-conjunctiva, respectively.

9.2.9   Putterman's Ptosis Clamp

Fig. 9.9 Putterman's
ptosis clamp

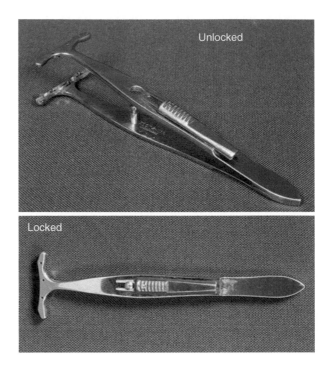

Key Features It is a specific instrument having two limbs with a slide lock on a superior limb. It has a horizontal wing-shaped clamp with three holes on the superior wing and three corresponding vertical pins over the inferior wing (Fig. 9.9). The front edge of the wing has a central concavity opposite central hole to expose the superior tarsal plate border maximally.

Uses
- Used in conjunctiva-Muller resection surgery for mild ptosis
- Can be used for the Fasanella-Servat procedure (Tarsal-conjunctiva-Muller resection)
- Can also be used in the conjunctival approach of levator resection (Blaskovics' operation)

Instrument Handling After double eversion of the upper eyelid, the central, medial, and lateral marking of conjunctiva toward superior fornix is done approximately 4 mm from the superior tarsal border (every 4 mm of resection corrects approximately 1–2 mm of ptosis). Then passing the retaining sutures from conjunctiva to skin, the conjunctiva is held taut at medial and lateral markings, and the Putterman's ptosis clamp is applied after closing and locking both limbs. Now the clamp is held horizontally, and a sharp blade/monopolar cautery tip is used to cut the tissues abutting the curved front edge of the clamp. The horizontal serrations and the three vertical pins provide sufficient holding effect to the tissues held inside the clamp. The application and removal of the clamp should be gentle to avoid any avulsion or abrasions to the soft tissues.

9.2.10 Wright's Ptosis Needle

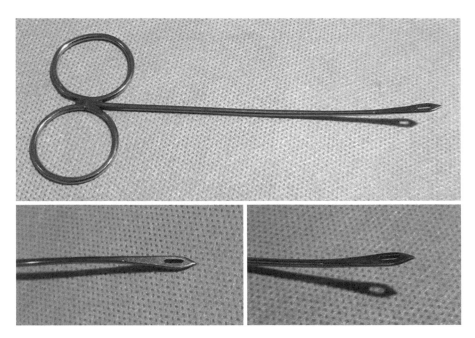

Fig. 9.10 Wright's ptosis needle

Key Features It is a long, sharp, and curved needle with an oval-/slit-shaped eyelet (1 × 6 mm) near its tip (Fig. 9.10). The sharp tip ensures smoother passage through soft tissues, while the eyelet is used to pass the edge of the fascia lata strip through it. It has a single or double ringed handle for holding and pulling it out.

Uses
- To pass the preserved or autologous fascia lata strips from one incision to other in frontalis sling suspension surgery
- To pass palmaris longus tendon strip or any synthetic suture material for similar surgery
- Can rarely be used to pass the transnasal wire for the correction of telecanthus

Instrument Handling After harvesting the fascia lata strips and fashioning the skin-muscle incisions, the Wright's ptosis needle is passed from one incision to the adjacent through the deep muscular plane. Minimal manipulations of the tract are recommended to have a straight path for the sling material. Once the needle tip and eyelet comes out, one end of the thin strip of fascia lata is passed through the eyelet and is retracted back via the primary entry site incision (railroad technique). Hence, fascia lata passage track is opposite to that of the ptosis needle. Utmost care is taken while passing the needle from eyebrow to the eyelid and vice versa as any misdirection, jerk, and extra force may lead to devastating globe penetration. To prevent it, these crucial passes should be made only when a Jaeger's eyelid plate guards the globe.

9.2.11 Crouch's Corneal Protector

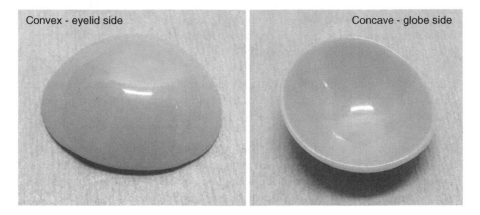

Convex - eyelid side

Concave - globe side

Fig. 9.11 Crouch's corneal protector

Key Points It is a hemispherical device with a diameter ranging from 18 to 26 mm. It is generally made up of medical-grade plastic, acrylic, or silicone, and the majority of inner concavity has a scleral base, while cornea remains contact-free (Fig. 9.11). Usually, it is a single-use item but can be cleaned appropriately and plasma sterilized for 2–3 uses.

Uses
- To protect cornea, sclera, and conjunctiva from instrument-related mechanical injuries
- To guard against the indirect conjunctival, corneal, or scleral damage with radio-frequency cautery tip or heat cautery
- Provides mechanical support while fashioning eyelid incisions
- Keeps the patient's vision occluded and prevents apprehension and anxiety

Instrument Handling The ocular surface should be properly anesthetized, and the cornea should be preferably covered with a viscoelastic agent or ointment to prevent surface abrasions. The corneal protector shell should be gently introduced, first into the superior fornix followed by gentle exposure of inferior fornix and sliding of the lower eyelid over the shell. This is a universal device and is of particular use in many eyelid surgeries. After the completion of surgery, it should be carefully and gently removed by first sliding the inferior edge out over the inferior eyelid. The superior portion generally slides out under the contraction effect of orbicularis oculi, but it can be taken out with the help of a toothed forceps if operated under general anesthesia. The forceps provides a firm grasp and prevents slippage. For residents and beginners, do not forget to remove it before starting the flap suturing in Cutler-Beard or Hughes' eyelid reconstruction procedure else it will be caught under both sutured eyelids. One should ensure the removal of shell from the first eye before proceeding onto the second. In rare situations, if the patient's eye is patched with the retained corneal protector, the patient might come after few hours of surgery with severe ocular pain/discomfort and foreign body sensation. One should always open the patch, examine and remove the protector, examine for corneal epithelial defects, and manage the situation, conservatively.

Specific wavelength (532 nm, 1064 nm) blocking protectors are also available which are used during the laser skin resurfacing or pigment reduction procedures for conditions like nevus of Ota and nevus flammeus.

Recent Trends The use of "silicone rod" in the frontalis sling suspension surgery has been accepted as most widely used material nowadays for the surgery in eyelids having blepharoptosis with poor levator action. A new sophisticated instrument called as Crawford's fascia lata stripper is also used for harvesting a longer length of fascia lata through a small incision over the thigh. It has a metered scale which leads to a relatively accurate length of the harvested fascia lata without increasing the length of the skin wound. The use of endoscope has also been used to provide a longer length of fascia lata for the frontalis sling suspension surgery.

Suggested Reading

1. Dave TV, Sharma P, Nayak A, Moharana R, Naik MN. Outcomes of frontalis sling versus levator resection in patients with monocular elevation deficiency associated ptosis. Ophthalmic Plast Reconstr Surg. 2018; https://doi.org/10.1097/IOP.0000000000001221.
2. Stump M, McConnell LK, Chahal HS, Shriver EM. Oculoplastic Basic Instrument Tray. EyeRounds.org. March 13, 2017. Available from: http://eyerounds.org/tutorials/instruments/Oculoplastics/OculoplasticTray/index.htm.

Instruments for Enucleation and Evisceration

10

Manpreet Singh, Prerana Tahiliani, and Varshitha Hemanth

10.1 Introduction

Enucleation involves removal of the entire globe, with preservation of all other peri-orbital and orbital structures. Evisceration involves removal of the ocular contents from an intact sclera, and exenteration refers to removal of the entire orbital contents, including the globe and soft tissues.

A thorough preoperative ophthalmic work-up, imaging (ultrasound B-scan and/or CT/MRI scan)—to note the presence of an intraocular tumor/extent of the tumor—written informed consent mentioning the laterality or side in bold letters (**Right**, **OD** or **Left**, **OS**), consultation by two ophthalmologists, marking of the eye (preoperative), and pupillary dilatation stand vital in the preparation of surgery. Before the first incision, the surgeon should ensure that the correct eye is going to be operated by an indirect-ophthalmoscopic examination.

M. Singh (✉)
Oculoplastics Services, Department of Ophthalmology, Advanced Eye Centre, Post Graduate Institute of Medical Education and Research (PGIMER), Chandigarh, India

P. Tahiliani
Oculoplastics and Ocular Oncology, Mumbai Eye Plastic Surgery, Mumbai, India

V. Hemanth
Clinical Fellow in Ophthalmic Plastic Surgery, Ocular Oncology and Socket Sciences, L V Prasad Eye Institute (LVPEI), Hyderabad, India

© Springer Nature Singapore Pte Ltd. 2019
P. Ichhpujani, M. Singh (eds.), *Ophthalmic Instruments and Surgical Tools*,
Current Practices in Ophthalmology,
https://doi.org/10.1007/978-981-13-7673-3_10

10.2   Instrumentation

10.2.1   Wells Enucleation Spoon

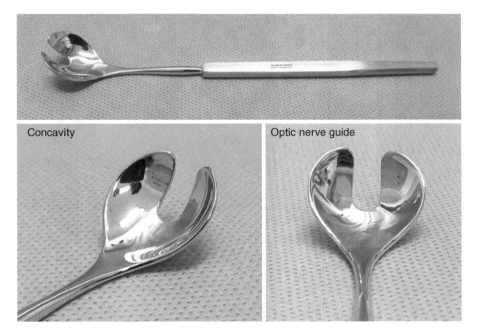

Fig. 10.1   Wells enucleation spoon

Key Features   It has a spoonlike, shallow, concave, hemispherical end attached to a long shaft (Fig. 10.1). The spoon is available in 15–21 mm diameter for phthisical or staphylomatous globes, to provide proper grip and contain the posterior portion of the eyeball. It features an optic nerve guide or groove (10 × 5 mm) for the engagement of the optic nerve.

Uses
- To perform enucleation in advanced malignant intraocular tumors not amenable for focal or local therapy (retinoblastoma, uveal melanoma)
- To perform enucleation while harvesting an eyeball during an "eye donation"
- To enucleate an eye with phthisis bulbi for cosmetic rehabilitation (posttraumatic, congenital partial anophthalmia)
- To perform therapeutic enucleation for painful blind eyes

Instrument Handling   Always confirm the laterality of the eye to be enucleated. A retrobulbar injection of 2% lignocaine + 0.5% bupivacaine mixed with 1:100,000 adrenaline provides sufficient anesthesia and akinesia. This negates the pain;

intraoperative hemorrhage prevents oculocardiac reflex and reduces postoperative pain. Hence it is beneficial for the patients under GA, too. Retrobulbar anesthesia also displaces the eyeball forward making it surgically more accessible. After tagging the recti and cutting them from the globe, the enucleation spoon is passed laterally, keeping the concavity up toward the globe. The plane should be between the isolated lateral rectus and the globe. The optic nerve is felt with the edge of the spoon and is guided into the dedicated groove. Now, the globe is lifted with an outward pulling force which stretches the intraorbital part of the optic nerve. The pulling force should be just less than to cause corneal edema. Then, the optic nerve is incised or cut with scissors, while the globe rests safely inside the spoon due to attached oblique muscles and soft tissue.

Rarely, with an excessive force, the intracanalicular portion of the optic nerve can be pulled into the orbit, and if incised near the orbital apex, the cut end of ophthalmic artery may retract back into the bony optic canal or brain and may lead to intracerebral hemorrhage. Hence, the pull and cut of optic nerve should be titrated appropriately. *Caution*—proper care should be taken not to cause any inadvertent penetration of globe and conversion of intraocular to an extraocular/orbital intraocular tumor.

10.2.2 Metzenbaum or Storz Enucleation Scissors

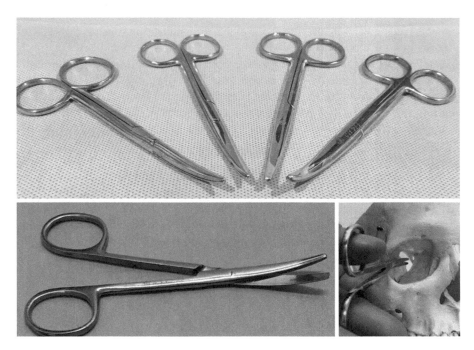

Fig. 10.2 Metzenbaum or Storz enucleation scissors

Key Features This scissors have 40–44 mm long, stout, broad, and curved blades with blunt tips (Fig. 10.2). The length provides good access to the optic nerve near orbital apex, blunt tips taking care not to injure other vital orbital structures and broad/stout blades delivering adequate force to cut optic nerve. The ring handles help in firm hold and application of force. The lap joint facilitates proper cleaning.

Uses
- Used primarily to perform cutting of optic nerve during an enucleation
- Can be used to carry out blunt dissection around orbital mass lesions
- Can be used to perform full-thickness eyelid incisions or lateral canthotomy in emergency situations
- Can be used to cut thick cotton/gauze pieces, thin drain pipes, etc.
- Can be used to perform tenotomy if appropriate scissors are not available

Instrument Handling After securing and pulling the globe with Wells enucleation spoon, the scissors are held firmly in the thumb and index finger of the dominant hand. The closed tip of scissors is guided into the orbital cavity between the shaft of the enucleation spoon and secured lateral rectus muscle. Now, the optic nerve is first "felt" with the closed tip of scissors. After feeling the optic nerve (firm cord-like), gentle strumming movements are performed to have an idea about its location and thickness and to create some space around the optic nerve. After localizing the optic nerve, the blades of scissors are opened gently to engage the optic nerve, and a single, bold cut is executed. Adrenaline-soaked gauze is kept ready before this step to pack the intraconal space immediately as this step prevents bleeding and hematoma collection. Following these steps prevents the multiple, desperate, and traumatic failed attempts to cut the optic nerve, resulting in various inadvertent injuries to the surrounding cranial nerves and blood vessels traversing the superior orbital fissure.

10.2.3 Mule and Bunge Evisceration Scoop

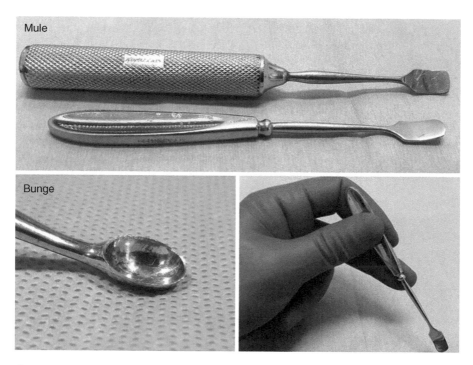

Fig. 10.3 Mule and Bunge evisceration scoop

Key Points Mule evisceration scoop has a thick/broad handle for firm grip; the business end has a stout, curved, and spatulated scoop (Fig. 10.3). The forward edge of the scoop is blunt, tapered, and curved to follow the inner scleral curvature. The overall length of this multipurpose instrument is 125–130 mm.

Uses
- To scoop out the majority of uveal tissue and other intraocular contents during an evisceration
- To scrape off the residual uveal tissue from the posterior inner scleral surface
- To perform blunt dissection around orbital masses
- To scoop out well-defined orbital lesion/masses
- Can be used a soft tissue retractor in orbitotomy procedures
- Can be used a platform/guard to fashion small eyelid, canthal incisions

Instrument Handling After performing a 360° conjunctival-limbal peritomy, the corneal button is removed. Now, a plane is created between the ciliary body and sclera and is extended 360° with a Barraquer or Castroviejo cyclodialysis spatula. Then, the evisceration scoop is passed in this plane from the scleral edge and moved till the posterior-most sclera. Now, the scoop is moved 360° in a circular motion to dissect the uvea from the sclera, posteriorly. Ideally, all the intraocular contents, i.e., uvea, retina, and vitreous, should be scooped out in a single attempt, and all specimens should be sent for histopathology. Sometimes one may require multiple attempts to remove the adherent; finer uveal tissue tags completely from the sclera with the help of smaller spatulas, especially from the vortex vein sites. Some surgeons use 95% ethanol application on the inner side of the scleral cavity for the complete destruction of the uveal pigment before inserting an intrascleral implant. The shape of Bunge evisceration scoop helps in the removal of adherent uveal tissue.

10.2.4 Castroveijo Cyclodialysis Spatula

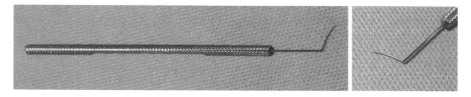

Fig. 10.4 Castroveijo cyclodialysis spatula

Key Features It is a 13.3 cm long, double-ended instrument with very fine slightly curved flat blades (15 × 0.5 mm, 10 × 0.5 mm) (Fig. 10.4). This is a universal instrument; the curved flat blades have blunt tips and edges for atraumatic insertion and manipulations.

Uses
- To initiate and create a cleft or plane between the sclera and ciliary body during an evisceration procedure
- Can rarely be used in place of iris repositor
- Can also be used to release the posterior iris-lens synechiae
- To release the secondary adhesion of iris with intraocular lens
- In the past, used to perform cyclodialysis (a surgical procedure for glaucoma)

Instrument Handling After removing the corneal button, the scleral edge is held by a toothed forceps, and the blunt tip of cyclodialysis spatula is gently teased between the sclera and ciliary body. During this, the convexity of the spatula is always kept outward which matches the inner curvature of the scleral cavity. Once the whole length is introduced between the desired plane, a 360° rotation of the instrument is carried out for the anterior separation of the uveal tissue from the sclera. While performing any intraocular movement with this instrument, always keep the curvature of the spatula in mind.

10.2.5 Disposable Orbital Implant Introducer

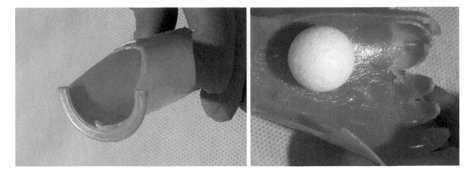

Fig. 10.5 Disposable orbital implant introducer

Key Features This plastic instrument has multiple, curved flanges at the business end and a border/stem for holding during the implant insertion (Fig. 10.5). It conforms into a funnel-like shape when scrolled for its easier insertion.

Uses
- To introduce the dense porous polyethylene implant in the intraconal cavity
- To introduce the PMMA implant into the desired location
- Provides better and smoother insertion for the implant wrapped with the sclera

Instrument Handling The inserter is scrolled into a funnel-like a shape and held in similar form for insertion. The intraconal space is exposed by holding the inter-muscular sheath with non-toothed forceps. The conical configuration helps in the insertion of the introducer into the desired location (intraconal) and depth of the orbit. Once inserted, it is kept stable in position with left hand; the implant is held and placed into the funnel safely, to prevent it from popping out. The implant is pushed with the tip of index finger or thumb of right hand, to the desired depth. The thumb or finger should not be pulled out at any point to prevent any back prolapse of the implant. Keeping the finger and implant in position, the edge of the inserter is grasped with the left hand and pulled out of orbit, slowly and gradually. Application of ointment on inner margins of the flanges helps in more comfortable slippage of the implant out of the inserter.

10.2.6 Carter Sphere Holder and Introducer

Fig. 10.6 Carter sphere
holder and introducer

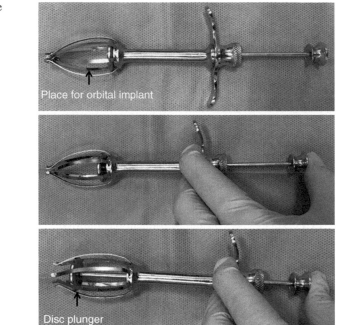

Key Features It has petal-shaped, long, metal flanges, with out-flared ends. The proximal broad/wide cavity is for holding an orbital implant; a disc plunger with a spring loading action pushes the implant, while the ringed handle provides stability to the instrument (Fig. 10.6). It is a good alternative to disposable plastic inserter at high-volume centers.

Uses
- To introduce any orbital implant safely into the desired intraconal compartment
- For easier insertion and accurate placement of an implant in a contracted or a posttraumatic socket
- For accurately placing a customized orbital prosthesis or anteriorly/partially sclera-coated porous implants

Instrument Handling The orbital implant is loaded safely inside the petals of the inserter in the desired orientation with the anterior surface toward the plunger side. Hence, the posterior surface of the implant will be pushed first into the orbital cavity. After loading the implant, the intraconal orbital space is adequately exposed. The inserter is held stable in the index and middle finger of the dominant hand, while the thumb is placed over the plunger head. Now, the flanged tips are gently introduced into the intraconal orbital space, and the implant is pushed into the cavity with a constant force. The spherical implant pushes open the flanges while maintaining its alignment, and once the equator of implant crosses the bent portion of flanges, the sphere gets a quick push into the orbital cavity. The inserter should be kept stable during this whole process for the proper placement of an implant at the appropriate depth. Care is taken while withdrawing the instrument to prevent the implant prolapse.

10.2.7 Foster Enucleation Snare

Fig. 10.7 Enucleation snare

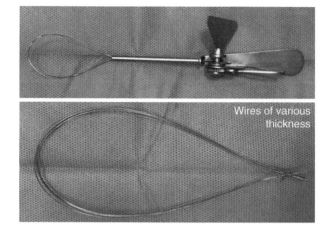

Wires of various thickness

Key Features This instrument consists of a fine, stainless steel wire (snare) passed as a loop through a slender and stout pipe (Fig. 10.7). The twisting of wing nut closes the loop, while the instrument is held stable by a strong handle.

Uses
- To perform enucleation in eyes where the longer optic nerve is necessary (e.g., retinoblastoma)
- To perform enucleation in small and contracted bony sockets

Instrument Handling The muscle stumps attached to the globe are secured with traction sutures for pulling the globe. Once the snare loop is passed over the sutures, it is gently teased over the equator of the globe (>25 mm diameter). Once it crosses the largest diameter of the eyeball, the snare is gently tightened and is pushed vertically downward over the length of the optic nerve to the desired depth into the orbit. The sliding of snare wire over the optic nerve can be helped with a forceps. Once the depth is reached, the snare is held firmly in non-dominant hand, while the wing nut is slowly twisted for tightening of the snare. A gentle "give way" feel provides the clue for optic nerve severance. The orbital cavity is packed quickly with adrenaline-soaked gauze piece to reduce bleeding which is rare in a snare enucleation. The globe is now pulled out and freed from the rest of adhesions.

Recent Trends Spherical or customized orbital implants made up of polymethylmethacrylate (PMMA), or dense porous polyethylene is used during the enucleation and evisceration surgeries to replace the volume loss. The implants are preferably covered in a scleral shell and placed inside the intraconal orbital space followed by the suturing of muscles and Tenon's capsule over it. The diameter of the orbital implant is calculated by measuring the axial length of opposite eyeball and reducing 2 mm from it. The placement of conformer at the end of surgery or in the early postoperative period is vital for the deepening of fornices followed by the placement of a customized ocular prosthesis.

Suggested Reading

1. Dave TV, Tiple S, Vempati S, Palo M, Ali MJ, Kaliki S, Naik MN. Low-cost three-dimensional printed orbital template-assisted patient-specific implants for the correction of spherical orbital implant migration. Indian J Ophthalmol. 2018;66(11):1600–7.
2. Mourits DL, Hartong DT, Bosscha MI, Kloos RJ, Moll AC. Worldwide enucleation techniques and materials for treatment of retinoblastoma: an international survey. PLoS One. 2015;10(3):e0121292.
3. Tyers AG. Evisceration, enucleation and exenteration. In: Medel R, Vásquez LM, editors. Orbital surgery. ESASO course series, vol. 5. Basel: Karger; 2014. p. 73–91.

Instruments Used in Orbital Surgeries

11

Manpreet Singh and Manpreet Kaur

11.1 Introduction

Orbital surgery deals with a variety of conditions involving the eye socket comprising of inflammatory diseases such as thyroid-associated orbitopathy, tumors, infections, and trauma. This chapter reviews the basic instruments used during orbital surgeries.

11.2 Instrumentation

Basics of Tissue Retraction for Orbital Surgeries: The orbital retractors are mainly used for keeping the orbital fat, muscles, eyeball, and other vital structures away from the operative field. The retraction is of utmost importance while working in deeper orbital cavities for a proper view of the delicate and vital anatomical structures.

After the incision over the skin, muscle, and orbital septum, the orbital retractor is applied by the surgeon in a correct plane and is then handed over to the assistant to provide a clear view and wider space and avoid injury to the surrounding vital structures. After that, the planned orbital mass removal, excision, or incision can be carried out. The assistant must remain alert while retracting during longer surgeries as a small inadvertent movement can lead to intraoperative

M. Singh (✉)
Oculoplastics Services, Department of Ophthalmology, Advanced Eye Centre, Post Graduate Institute of Medical Education and Research (PGIMER), Chandigarh, India

M. Kaur
Glaucoma Services, Department of Ophthalmology, Advanced Eye Centre, Post Graduate Institute of Medical Education and Research (PGIMER), Chandigarh, India

© Springer Nature Singapore Pte Ltd. 2019
P. Ichhpujani, M. Singh (eds.), *Ophthalmic Instruments and Surgical Tools*,
Current Practices in Ophthalmology,
https://doi.org/10.1007/978-981-13-7673-3_11

complications. The assistant is also advised to intermittently release the pressure from the eyeball or soft tissues to minimize the chances of a hypoxic/anoxic injury to the optic nerve. Moreover, the orbital retractors are extremely helpful during cauterization of a bleeder or a cryo application. During orbital floor repair, the retractors keep the extracted fat or muscle away from the fracture site to prevent entrapment until an implant sheet is not applied over the fracture.

11.2.1 Malleable Ribbon Retractors

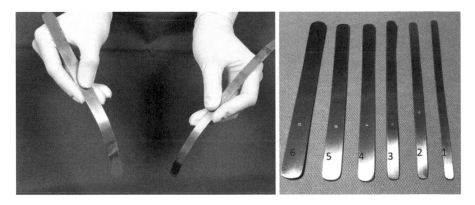

Fig. 11.1 Malleable ribbon retractors

Key Features These are long, ribbonlike, malleable strips of stainless steel. The length is around 15 cm for all, but the width ranges from 0.5 cm to 1.5 cm (Fig. 11.1). The edges are blunt and non-traumatic, and either business end has a rounded edge or oval configuration. The surface is made non-refractile to prevent intraoperative glare.

Uses
- To retract the eyeball, orbital fat, and lacrimal gland during orbitotomy surgeries.
- To retract the lifted periosteum and orbital fat during the orbital floor fracture repairs.
- To protect the eyeball during the usage of an oscillating saw or powered drill over the adjacent bones.
- To lift the skin and soft tissue while performing an endoscopic eyebrow lift, dermoid cyst removal, and endoscopic harvest of fascia lata.
- During orbital incisional biopsies, removal of orbital foreign bodies, and external orbital decompression surgery.

- Acts as a platform for cutting the small skin or mucosal grafts.
- Overall, this is a very versatile instrument which can be used in any kind of procedure as an adjunct.

Instrument Handling Being a flexible, ribbonlike flat instrument, it is easy to mold or modify the length and angle of the retractor, going in the orbit (Fig. 11.1). The assistant can also modify the length and angulation of the segment used to hold the retractor. Once the soft tissue dissection is complete, the blades of blunt-tipped Stevens tenotomy scissors are kept open inside the wound, and gently the tip of the retractor is introduced into the wound. Generally, the retraction forces are directed toward the soft tissue and away for bone. The assistant bent end should be angulated superiorly for the grip to be comfortable providing better stability and longer retraction without undue movements. The reinsertions and removals should be smooth and in sync with the surgeon. A broad 1–1.5 cm retractor is used to protect the globe while using powered instruments on the bone.

11.2.1.1   Helveston–Barbie Tissue Retractor

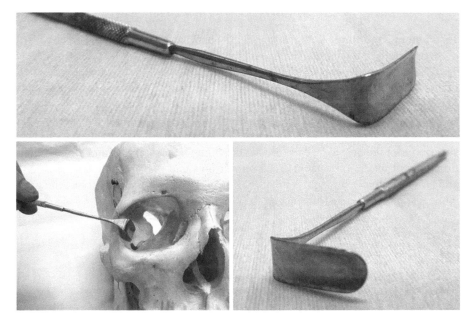

Fig. 11.2   Helveston–Barbie tissue retractor

Key Features   The retractor blade is approximately 6 cm long and 1 cm wide with a concavity along its width in the inferior half (Fig. 11.2). This concavity provides more extensive space for operating while simultaneously retracting the orbital tissues. The assistant arm is long and cylindrical and has a knurled surface for better grip during the retraction.

Uses
- To retract the eyeball, orbital fat, and lacrimal gland during orbitotomy surgeries.
- To retract the lifted periosteum and orbital fat during the orbital floor fracture repairs.
- To protect the eyeball during the usage of an oscillating saw or powered drill over the adjacent bones.
- To lift the skin and soft tissue while performing an endoscopic eyebrow lift, dermoid cyst removal, and endoscopic harvest of fascia lata.
- During orbital incisional biopsies, removal of orbital foreign bodies and external orbital decompression surgery.
- Acts as a platform for cutting the small skin or mucosal grafts.
- Overall, this is a very versatile instrument which can be used in any procedure as an adjunct.

11.2.1.2   Sewell Orbital Retractors

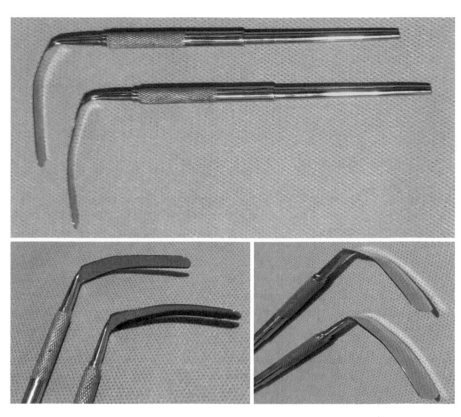

Fig. 11.3 Sewell orbital retractors

Key Points The stainless steel retractor blade has a concave, smooth inner surface which has a fixed angulation. It is attached to a straight cylindrical shaft with a knurled segment for better and longer grip (Fig. 11.3). The business end edge has a non-traumatic, rounded configuration.

Uses
- To retract the eyeball, orbital fat, and lacrimal gland during orbitotomy surgeries
- To retract the lifted periosteum and orbital fat during the orbital floor fracture repairs
- To protect the eyeball during the usage of an oscillating saw or powered drill over the adjacent bones
- To lift the skin and soft tissue while performing an endoscopic eyebrow lift, dermoid cyst removal, and endoscopic harvest of fascia lata
- During orbital incisional biopsies, removal of orbital foreign bodies and external orbital decompression surgery

Instrument Handling As most of the retractors are held and used, similar principles apply to this instrument. The longer length of the blades can be of some disadvantage for anterior surgical areas but serves a vital role for the deeper orbital surgeries like optic canal decompression, etc.

11.2.1.3 Schepens Retractor

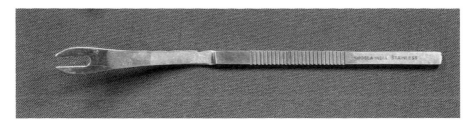

Fig. 11.4 Schepens retractor

Key Points A 14 × 61-mm-long slender instrument with a forked business end for facilitating the passage of the needle of the suture (Fig. 11.4). It provides better identification of a bleeding vessel and can make the target area more prominent.

Uses
- To retract the eyeball and identify the desired scleral region for passing the Dacron sutures in a scleral buckling surgery
- Can also be used during an anterior orbitotomy and orbital foreign body removal procedure

Instrument Handling All orbital retractors have long blades but may have variable widths (6–17 mm) and shapes. The blunt edges and concave or flat surfaces are also common features.

- Helveston–Barbie retractor has smaller, less curved blades as compared to Sewell and has variable widths of 7, 9, and 11 mm.
- The Sewell retractors set contains long blades with different widths and knurled handles for better grasp to prevent slippage during long orbital surgeries.

11.2.2 Screws and Orbital Plates

Straight and angled plates for orbital fracture repair

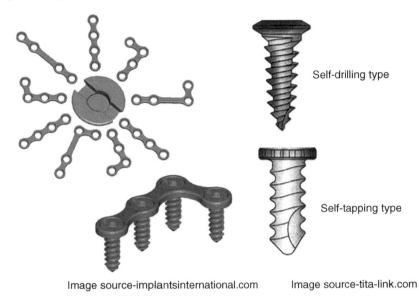

Self-drilling type

Self-tapping type

Image source-implantsinternational.com   Image source-tita-link.com

Fig. 11.5 Straight and angled plates. Self-drilling and self-tapping type of cortical screws. (Source: implantsinternationbal.com and tita-link.com)

Key Features The cortical screws come in two variants: self-tapping (constant diameter of the whole shaft) and self-drilling (tapering diameter for easier entry and progress) (Fig. 11.5). The screw heads have two configurations, cross-drive and hexa-drive, depending upon the number of edges. Depending upon these, the screwdrivers blades with holding devices are available in similar cross-drive and hexa-drive pattern. Their length varies from 3 mm to 9 mm, and 4–6 mm is the routinely used ones. Usually, there are five pieces per pack. The steel, titanium, or gold orbital plates vary from 0.25 mm to 0.3 mm thickness and are available in various configurations, but the straight and curved are commonly used for orbital procedures. They usually range from 2, 4, 6, 8, 10, 14, to 18 holes depending upon the size and site of the fracture.

Uses
- To fix and stabilize the fractured and displaced bones of the orbital rim
- To stabilize the bones of a tripod fracture
- To fix the orbital floor implant (titanium, etc.) to the orbital rim

Instrument Handling After putting the desired shape and size of the orbital floor or orbital rim implant, the type of plate and the locations of the screws are determined and marked. The screws, self-drilling type or self-tapped, are loaded onto the self-retaining screwdriver directly from the screw containing plate and are tightened for better screwing efficiency and stability. The drilling if needed is performed with utmost care avoiding the bone-burn and consequential screw loosening or infection. The screwdriver is always kept stable, and the screw can be pushed vertically or obliquely depending upon the thickness of the available bone in the region. The endpoint is neither too tight or too loose, and the bevel of the head should engage in the plate hole for best possible stability.

Recent Trends The porous polyethylene sheets and titanium meshes are being used in the repair of orbital floor or wall fractures. The porous polyethylene sheets can have one side porous (tissue ingrowth) and other nonporous (no tissue ingrowth). The nonporous side is kept toward orbital fat and extraocular muscles to prevent restriction of eye movements. The porous nature allows the ingrowth of fibrovascular tissue for better scaffold-like action in more natural way. Orbital rim implants and subperiosteal implants are also used in specific cases. Customized 3-D reconstructed models made with 3-D printers are also used for difficult cases.

Suggested Reading

1. Khorasani M, Janbaz P, Rayati F. Maxillofacial reconstruction with Medpor porous polyethylene implant: a case series study. J Korean Assoc Oral Maxillofac Surg. 2018;44(3):128–35.
2. Rai A, Datarkar A, Arora A, Adwani DG. Utility of high density porous polyethylene implants in maxillofacial surgery. J Maxillofac Oral Surg. 2014;13(1):42–6.
3. Szymor P, Kozakiewicz M. Modification of orbital retractor to facilitate the insertion of orbital wall implants. Br J Oral Maxillofac Surg. 2017;55(6):633–4.

Common Instruments Used in Refractive Surgeries

12

Monika Balyan, Chintan Malhotra, and Arun K. Jain

12.1 Introduction

Refractive surgeries are performed with the aim of decreasing or eliminating dependency on glasses or contact lenses. These include various methods of surgical reshaping of the cornea (keratomileusis), implantation of phakic intraocular lenses (IOLs) or clear lens extractions with IOL implantation.

Corneal surgeries may be divided into the following.

12.1.1 'Flap'- and 'Cap'-Based Procedures

- **Laser-assisted in situ keratomileusis (LASIK)**: Femtosecond laser or a mechanical microkeratome is used to create a partial-thickness lamellar corneal flap with a small uncut area known as the 'hinge'. After lifting the flap, a 193 nm argon fluoride excimer laser is used to ablate the stromal bed following which the flap is repositioned.
- **Refractive lenticule extraction (ReLEx)**: ReLEx 'FLEx' (femtosecond lenticule extraction): A femtosecond laser cuts a lenticule within the corneal stroma. Afterwards, a LASIK-like flap is cut which can be lifted to access the lenticule and flap repositioned. This procedure has now been replaced by ReLEx SMILE.
- **ReLEx 'SMILE'** (small incision lenticule extraction): A femtosecond laser is used to create an intrastromal lenticule between two photodisruption planes at approximately 120–140 microns depth (the 'cap') from the surface. This lenticule is extracted via a 2–3 mm arcuate side cut.

M. Balyan · C. Malhotra (✉) · A. K. Jain
Cataract and Refractive Services, Department of Ophthalmology, Advanced Eye Centre,
Post Graduate Institute of Medical Education and Research (PGIMER), Chandigarh, India

© Springer Nature Singapore Pte Ltd. 2019
P. Ichhpujani, M. Singh (eds.), *Ophthalmic Instruments and Surgical Tools*,
Current Practices in Ophthalmology,
https://doi.org/10.1007/978-981-13-7673-3_12

12.1.2 Surface Procedures

Excimer laser is used to ablate the anterior corneal stroma in these procedures after removal of the epithelium, without creation of a stromal flap. The procedures differ in the way the epithelium is handled.

- **Photorefractive keratectomy (PRK):** The epithelium is debrided using alcohol followed by excimer laser surface ablation.
- **Epi-LASIK:** An epithelial flap with a hinge is created mechanically using a modified microkeratome with a dull blade and thin applanation plate, with the flap being repositioned back at the end of the excimer laser procedure.
- **Laser-assisted subepithelial keratomileusis (LASEK):** Also known as 'alcohol-assisted flap PRK', the epithelium is not debrided but is loosened with dilute alcohol, lifted like a flap with a hinge and then repositioned after excimer laser ablation.

12.1.3 Intraocular Procedures

These may be categorized into two major categories:

- Phakic intraocular lens (PIOL) implantation: e.g. Implantable Collamer Lenses (ICL™)
- Clear lens extraction

12.2 Instruments

A variety of instruments with modifications to the basic design are available for different refractive surgeries. Some of the more commonly used prototypes are described below.

12.2.1 Lid Speculum for Exposure

A good speculum providing adequate globe exposure is the foremost requirement for any refractive procedure to be done effectively.

Lieberman Temporal Speculum This is a self-retaining K-wire speculum with Kratz style open blades, and amount of the exposure required can be adjusted using a thumb screw control (Fig. 12.1). This also comes with a modification which incorporates silicon aspiration tubing to keep the interface debris free.

Fig. 12.1 Lieberman
temporal speculum

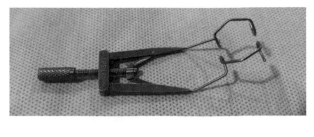

Fig. 12.2 Moria
Evolution 3E control unit

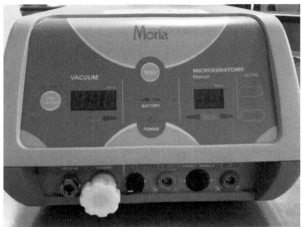

12.2.2 Instruments for Laser-Assisted In Situ Keratomileusis (LASIK)

12.2.2.1 Instruments for Flap Creation

a) **Microkeratome-assisted LASIK flap:** Creation of a LASIK flap with a micro-keratome requires a powered microkeratome cutting head and suction rings to stabilize the eye and generate vacuum. The microkeratome head has a highly sharpened cutting blade which should be discarded after each patient and an applanation head or plate which flattens the cornea in advance of the cutting blade. The cutting head usually attaches to a powered handpiece (motor) which may be electrical or gas driven and oscillates the blade at high speeds. The same or another motor also mechanically advances the cutting head across the cornea on the suction ring fixed to the globe. As an example the Moria Evolution 3E control unit along with its attachments is described below.

1. **Moria Evolution 3E control unit**
   This console operates the One Use-Plus, M2 Single-Use, Epi-K™ and the ALTK-CBm Systems (Fig. 12.2). It features two pumps to maintain a safe vacuum and two motors, one for head advancement and the other for blade oscillations with no oscillation on reverse movement. Two different translational speed settings are available. The slower (speed 1) of the two available speeds is recommended for the steeper and thinner corneas.

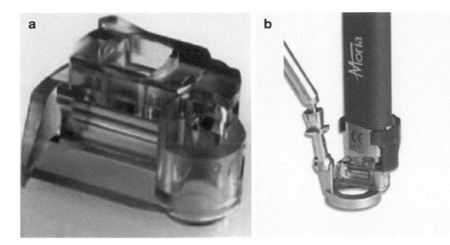

Fig. 12.3 (**a**) Moria M2 single-use head. (**b**) The head-suction ring assembly

2. **Mechanical microkeratomes**

- *Microkeratomes with rotational (pivotal) movement*

M2 Single-Use System This unit comprises an automated microkeratome with rotational movement available in different head sizes (90 and 130) for customization of the flap thickness (Fig. 12.3). The cutting mechanism consists of a blade in a disposable preassembled head, the advancement rate is adjustable, oscillation rate is 15,000 rpm, and the eye is fixated with suction rings of different sizes depending on the keratometry. A variable flap orientation is achievable with a 360° hinge position. The average flap thickness achieved with the 90 μm and 130 μm heads is 110 μm and 150 μm, respectively.

The Hansatome microkeratome by Bausch and Lomb is another example of a rotational microkeratome and produces a superiorly hinged flap.

- *Microkeratome with linear (translational) movement*

One Use-Plus SBK System This comprises an automated microkeratome with a linear movement and creates a flap with a nasal hinge (Fig. 12.4). Similar to the M2 single use, it has variable head sizes of 90 μm, 110 μm and 130 μm depth for altering the flap thickness and customizable flap sizes depending on the size of the suction rings chosen. The flaps created with this linear microkeratome have been shown to be more planar with greater predictability in the flap thickness achieved as compared to other mechanical microkeratomes.

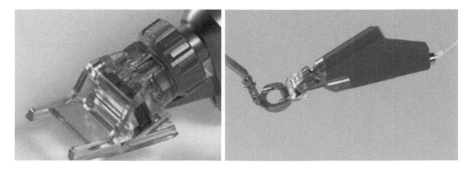

Fig. 12.4 Moria SBK microkeratome head, assembled blade and suction ring

Fig. 12.5 Suction ring for microkeratome LASIK

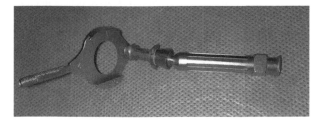

3. **Suction rings**

   These adhere to the globe and raise the intraocular pressure (IOP) to high levels for proper and safe cutting of the corneal flap (Fig. 12.5). Additionally they provide a stable platform for the movement of the microkeratome. The suction rings are connected to a vacuum pump, which is controlled by an on-off foot pedal. The rings are available in various sizes, e.g. 7.5, 8, 8.5 and 9 and have adjustable stops to change the size of the stabilizing hinge. The dimension of the suction ring determines the diameter of the flap. The size of the suction ring, hinge size and the speed of the blade can be adjusted depending on the patients' keratometry and white-to-white corneal diameter according to the nomogram provided by the manufacturer.

b) **Femtosecond laser-assisted LASIK flaps:** The flap creation with a femtosecond laser requires placement of a suction ring centred on the pupil followed by docking, keeping the suction ring parallel to the eye. An applanating glass lens (patient interface) is used to flatten the cornea (Fig. 12.6a) to ensure efficient delivery of the laser beam into the ocular tissues by optical coupling and to stabilize the globe. In some systems, a suction ring is placed around the limbus first, and then the applanation cone is docked into it (e.g. IntraLase iFS 150 kHz by Abbott Medical Optics Inc., Santa Ana, California) (Fig. 12.6b), while others have suction ring coupled to the applanation cone (VisuMAX by Carl Zeiss Meditec AG, Jena, Germany) (Fig. 12.6c). The shape of the applanation interface can be planar (IntraLase), modified planar (WaveLight FS 200 by Alcon Laboratories Inc., Ft Worth, Texas) or curved (VisuMAX).

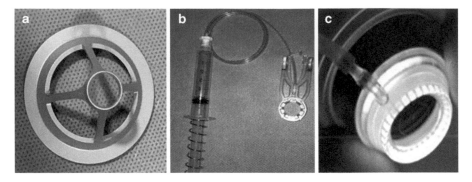

Fig. 12.6 Planar applanation cone (patient interface) with suction ring in IntraLase iFS 150 by AMO; (**b**): suction ring with syringe. (**c**) Curved patient interface in VisuMAX

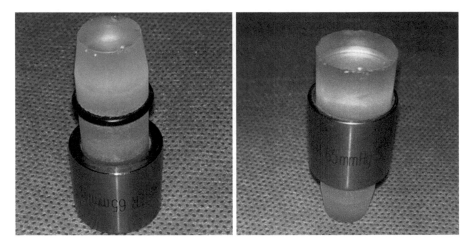

Fig. 12.7 Barraquer Applanation Tonometer

c) **Applanation tonometer**: In making LASIK flaps with mechanical microkeratomes, the applanation tonometer is utilized to check that an adequately high
   intraocular pressure has been achieved after activation of suction and prior to
   passing the microkeratome over the corneal surface. This is an essential step in
   order to minimize the risk of flap complications like thin or buttonholed flaps or
   inadvertent ocular perforation during the microkeratome pass.

Barraquer Applanation Tonometer

Based on the Maklakov's principle of applanation tonometry (constant force with
variable area), this tonometer consists of a conical shaft of high-density transparent
plastic, a silicone retaining ring and a slip ring handle (Fig. 12.7). Each tonometer
is identified as to mmHg on the anterior surface, while the flat applanating surface
is marked with two closely etched rings corresponding to the range of calibrated
intraocular pressure (IOP). On the tonometer used for microkeratome-assisted
LASIK, these rings correspond to an IOP range of 60–65 mmHg.

Prior to placing the flat applanating surface on the cornea, any excessive fluid on the cornea should be dried. After the eye is adequately pressurized, the tonometer is gently lowered onto the cornea till the slip ring allows the plastic tonometer to slide up. At this point the applanation can be seen through the tonometer. If the applanation is a small ring which does not fill within the etched rings, then the intraocular pressure is above the calibrated IOP. Conversely if the applanation circle goes beyond the range, the eye is too soft leading to excessive applanation by the tonometer.

12.2.2.2   Flap Markers

Different designs with variable marking patterns are available. Most of the instruments have a central optical zone to ensure proper centration over the flap. The marking is done using a gentian violet marker before lifting the flap. In routine cases, the markings help in accurate realignment of the edges of the flaps and guards against inadvertent flap folds. In situations with free caps, these markers act as a guide to prevent the flaps being placed upside down. The asymmetric marking patterns are especially helpful in the latter situation.

Culbertson LASIK Flap Marker

This has a round handle and five smooth-edged asymmetric markings for the proper repositioning of the flap (Fig. 12.8). It can be used for nasal as well as superior hinge locations. The marker is placed such that half the length of the individual limbs marks the upper surface of the flap, while the other half marks the corneal surface beyond the edges of the flap.

12.2.2.3   Spatulas for Elevating the Flap

Elevator spatulas are insinuated at the side cut close to the hinge on one side and advanced between the overlying flap and the underlying stromal bed to the opposite side cut. Depending on the superior or nasal location of the hinge, they are then swept either downwards or temporally, respectively, in a single or multiple sweeps.

a. **Seibel Flap Lifter and Retreatment Spatula**

Designed for lifting flaps created with the femtosecond laser as well as retreatment of any flaps, this is a double-ended spatula with a Z-shaped long tip at one end and a smaller tip at the other (Fig. 12.9). The tips are pointed to facilitate easy entry underneath the flap and to avoid trauma to the flap edges. The small tip can be used to initiate the separation at the periphery followed by inserting the longer tip in a gentle sweeping manner. The flap can then be lifted using the

Fig. 12.8 Culbertson LASIK flap marker

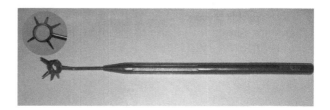

Fig. 12.9 Seibel flap lifter
and retreatment spatula

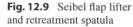
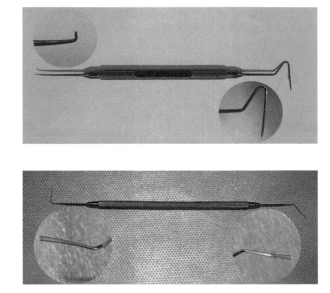

Fig. 12.10 LASIK flap
elevator

longer tip. Its design enables it to be used with a central pivoting technique, and it also minimizes the inherent torque which may be seen with conventional flap lifters. Care should be taken to avoid excessive force while using the long tip in cases of femto flaps which are tightly adherent as this can result in buttonholing of the flaps or damage to the underlying stroma.

b. **Double-Ended LASIK Flap Elevator**
This spatula may be used for lifting the created microkeratome flap as well as repositioning it after excimer ablation. The spatulated portions of the instrument are vaulted to conform to the natural curvature of the cornea. Each end has a rounded anterior surface, a flat posterior surface and a 2 mm rounded, slightly bevelled tip for entering through the peripheral edge of the flap before planar separation of the interface (Fig. 12.10).

12.2.2.4　Irrigation Cannulas

Cannulas are used to irrigate the interface and clear it of debris and epithelial cells before repositioning of the flap. They come in different shapes and sizes with different opening sites. These are designed to enter the interface with ease and have a smooth tip to avoid any trauma to the flap or the underlying stromal bed.

a. **Flattened cannula**
A disposable 27 G cannula with four ports at the side and an angulated curved anterior portion to aid ease of insertion can irrigate both sides of the flap at the same time (Fig. 12.11).

Fig. 12.11 Flattened
cannula

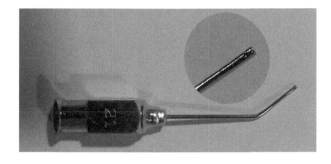

Fig. 12.12 Buratto
LASIK cannula

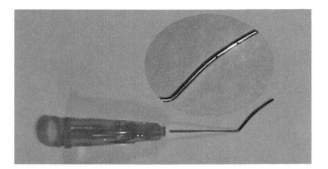

Fig. 12.13 Mendez
multipurpose LASIK
forceps

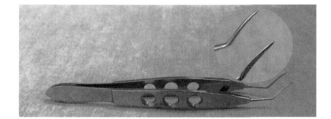

b. **Buratto LASIK cannula**

The cannula comes with a single small front and two larger side ports which are designed for equal flow in three directions (Fig. 12.12). It provides irrigation in multiple directions at the same time.

12.2.2.5   Forceps

Mendez Multipurpose LASIK Forceps

It has vaulted (12 mm long) shanks, spatulated jaws and tips along with smooth grasping surfaces (Fig. 12.13). It is used for lifting, dissecting and grasping the corneal flap.

Fig. 12.14 Buratto flap
protector

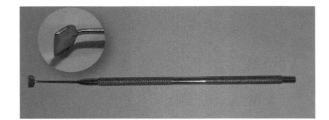

Fig. 12.15 Mannis-
Buratto flap protector

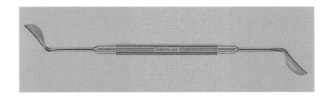

Fig. 12.16 Sri Ganesh
globe fixation forceps

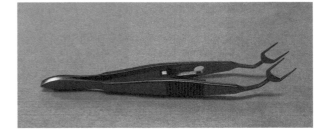

12.2.2.6   Flap Protectors
a. **Buratto Flap Protector**
   This instrument consists of a thin, convex blade angled at 45° with a narrow lip
   to positively engage and shield the nasally hinged flap during excimer laser ablation (Fig. 12.14). The edge of the spatula is positioned along the corneal flap
   hinge once it is everted. It prevents inadvertent exposure of the LASIK flap to the
   excimer laser which can induce irregular astigmatism.

b. **Mannis-Buratto Flap Protector**
   This is a double-ended instrument with blades angled at 15 degrees and is used
   to engage and protect superiorly hinged flaps (Fig. 12.15).

12.2.3 Instruments for Small Incision Lenticule
Extraction (SMILE)

1. **Globe Fixation Forceps:** These help in steady fixation of the globe. The widely
   spaced non-traumatic jaws allow fixation at two points, thus limiting tangential
   rotation, e.g. Sri Ganesh globe fixation forceps (Fig. 12.16). The lock ensures
   easy transfer from one hand to the other hand without causing much trauma.

2. **SMILE Lenticule Dissectors and Lifters**

These double-ended instruments usually have a smaller fine straight tip on one end and a longer smooth spoon shaped tip on the other end, e.g. Advance Chansue ReLEx dissector and lifter, Reinstein lenticule separator and Grewal Dissector and Lifter (Fig. 12.17). The small tip is used to open the incision followed by insertion of the longer end inside with the convexity facing down. With gentle swiping and back-forth movements, the lenticule is separated in two planes and hooked out using the spoon or grabbed with forceps. The surgeon strips the anterior surface first followed by the posterior surface, as inadvertent stripping of posterior surface first causes the lenticule to stick to the cap which may result in incomplete lenticule removal.

3. **Lenticule Extraction Forceps**

These forceps usually have curved shafts for easy manipulation between corneal planes, delicate serrated jaws and a blunt tip to allow for easy lenticule removal, e.g. TAN forceps, ALHF SMILE forceps and Sri Ganesh lenticule-removing forceps. In some variants, the upper jaw at the tip is longer then lower jaw to facilitate easy lenticule removal (Fig. 12.18). Once the lenticule is totally separated in two planes using the dissector, any of these forceps can be used to grasp and pull the lenticule through the arcuate incision. After the lenticule is taken out, it should be checked for circularity to ensure complete removal.

Fig. 12.17 Grewal dissector and lifter

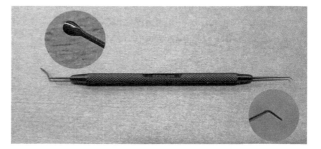

Fig. 12.18 SMILE lenticule extraction forceps with serrated jaws and blunt tips

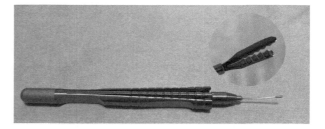

12.2.4 Instruments for LASEK and PRK

1. **LASEK Epithelial Trephine and Alcohol Retaining Well**
   This instrument has two ends with differing functions: one side has a 270° semi-sharp edge with a 90° cut out or two marks for the flap hinge and acts as an epithelial trephine, while the other end acts as a reservoir (well) for alcohol treatment to loosen the epithelium (Fig. 12.19). The well has dual fixation grooves to prevent leakage and stabilize the globe. It is usually 0.5 mm larger than the trephine to ensure penetration of the alcohol solution into the precut margin. The well is filled with 20% absolute alcohol for 20–30 s after placing it firmly on the cornea. The alcohol is then soaked up with Merocel sponges and the cornea irrigated thoroughly with balanced salt solution prior to epithelial debridement.

2. **Hockey Epithelial Removal Knife/PRK Spatula**
   This spatulated instrument has a thin smooth bottomed edge for gently scraping away the epithelium, while the spatula tip and top are slightly sharpened to facilitate more aggressive scraping. This spatula may be is used debridement of epithelium after alcohol treatment as well as for manual debridement (Fig. 12.20).

3. **LASEK Micro Hoe and Epi Peeler**
   The micro hoe has a contoured and angled face for precise resection of the edges of the adherent epithelium (Fig. 12.21). This instrument may be used for epithelial flap creation in LASEK or epithelial debridement in PRK. The other spatulated end has semi-sharp edges and can be used both for peeling back the central portion of the epithelial flap after the margin of the flap has been lifted and repositing back the flap after the procedure is complete.

Fig. 12.19 Epithelial trephine and alcohol well for PRK/LASEK

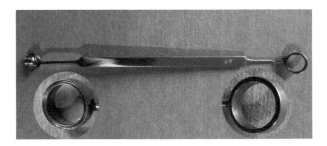

Fig. 12.20 Hockey epithelial removal knife

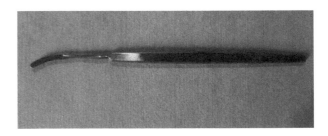

Fig. 12.21 LASEK micro hoe and epi peeler

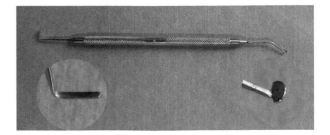

Fig. 12.22 Foam-tipped plunger

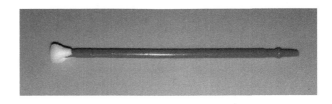

Fig. 12.23 ICL™ injector system with cartridge bay (inset)

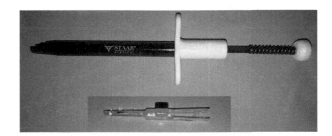

12.2.5 Instruments for Implantable Collamer Lens (ICL™) Implantation

1. **Foam-Tipped Plunger**
   This is used initially for picking the ICL from the container and placing it inside the cartridge bay (Fig. 12.22). The ball end of the plunger is later interlocked with the injector, and the foam tip is used to push the ICL inside the eye. It has to be ensured that the foam tip is hydrated as insufficient hydration may lead to trapping of the ICL between plunger and cartridge upon ICL delivery.

2. **ICL™ Injector System**
   This is a push mechanism spring-controlled injector which interlocks the foam-tipped plunger in its body, with the cartridge being inserted and locked into position at the anterior end (Fig. 12.23). The clear funnel of the cartridge (inset) allows for inspection under the microscope for proper orientation of the ICL.

3. **Forceps for ICL™ Lens**
   These coaxial 20 G forceps for loading of the ICL have an angled tip with smooth ridges for firmly grasping the ICL without damaging the optic of the lens

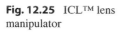

Fig. 12.24 Forceps for ICL™ lens

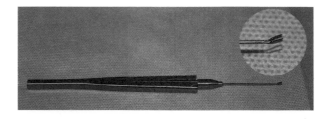

Fig. 12.25 ICL™ lens manipulator

(Fig. 12.24). The edge of the ICL is grasped with the forceps inserted through the nozzle end of the cartridge and pulled towards the nozzle tip. While pulling the ICL, the relative motion should be such that the hand holding the cartridge should be pulled away from the hand holding the forceps to prevent any damage to the ICL.

4. **ICL™ Lens Manipulator**

This instrument has a flat atraumatic olive-shaped tip to facilitate ICL manipulation inside the eye without causing any damage to the ICL, lens or the iris tissue (Fig. 12.25). It is used for positioning the ICL and nudging or tucking the ICL under the iris, into the sulcus. In cases of toric ICL, the instrument is used for rotation and axis alignment

Suggested Reading

1. https://www.ophthalmologyweb.com/Refractive/5251-Refractive-Surgery/

Refractive Surgery: Basics of Laser Consoles and Ablation Profiles

13

Aditi Mehta Grewal, Sartaj Singh Grewal, Anchal Thakur, Amit Gupta, and Chintan Malhotra

13.1 Introduction

Refractive procedures may be performed on the cornea or intraocularly. Laser-based corneal procedures broadly include photorefractive keratectomy (PRK), laser-assisted in situ keratomileusis (LASIK), refractive lenticule extraction (ReLEx), and small incision lenticule extraction (SMILE). While PRK and LASIK rely on excimer laser photoablation, ReLEx and SMILE are based on the photodisruptive femtosecond laser.

13.2 Laser-Tissue Interactions

LASER is an acronym for light amplification by stimulated emission of radiation. Three different types of laser-tissue interactions, i.e., photoablation, photodisruption, and photothermal, are applicable for laser refractive surgery.

A. M. Grewal · A. Thakur · A. Gupta · C. Malhotra (✉)
Cataract and Refractive Services, Department of Ophthalmology, Advanced Eye Centre,
Post Graduate Institute of Medical Education and Research (PGIMER), Chandigarh, India

S. S. Grewal
Grewal Eye Institute, Chandigarh, India

© Springer Nature Singapore Pte Ltd. 2019
P. Ichhpujani, M. Singh (eds.), *Ophthalmic Instruments and Surgical Tools*,
Current Practices in Ophthalmology,
https://doi.org/10.1007/978-981-13-7673-3_13

13.2.1 Photoablation

Photoablation involves breakage of chemical bonds with the help of excited dimers ("excimer"), most commonly the argon fluoride 193 nm excimer laser. Light emitted by this laser has high energy per photon, high precision, and a low tissue penetrance making it a safe laser for corneal refractive surgeries. By varying the ablation pattern, the excimer laser can alter the anterior corneal curvature to modify a particular refractive error.Structurally, the important parts of an excimer laser consist of:

- **Laser unit/laser cavity** consisting of a laser head with high-voltage power supply, a trigger unit, and a laser interface for generation of the laser radiation from the ArF mixture by an electric discharge.
- **Gas-handling system** which consists of laser gases (contained either in the two separate chambers to be mixed at a later stage or a premixed gas mixture ready for the reaction), a flushing gas (e.g., helium, nitrogen) which is flushed along the optic pathway to maintain its quality and cleanliness, valves, pressure sensors and reducers, vacuum pump, and filters.
- **Optical pathway** consisting of a complex array of lenses, mirrors, and prisms to homogenize the laser beam before it reaches the cornea.
- **Control panel** for control of distance lasers (to maintain correct height adjustment of the patients eye), white light illumination, and eye tracker parameters.
- **Eye tracker** to ensure alignment of the laser beam to the patient's eye.
- **Operating microscope** required during flap lifting, interface washing, and flap repositioning as well as to observe the patient's eye during the laser ablation. The illumination for the microscope head is provided by an array of light-emitting diodes (LEDs).
- **Plume removal system** – a blower and suction unit to ensure removal of debris and provide a controlled environment at the patient's eye.
- **Computer system** for data entry and for programming as well as regulation of the amount and pattern of energy to be delivered.
- **Motor-driven patient bed**
- Figure 13.1 shows the various parts of a fifth-generation excimer laser: the Mel 80 (Carl Zeiss Meditec AG, Jena, Germany).

13.2.1.1 Laser Beam Emission Systems
- **Broad beam:** These employ large diameter beams (7 mm) with slower repetition rates, very high energy per pulse beam, and therefore a fewer number of pulses. The corneal tissue is removed layer by layer. While earlier lasers suffered from the side effects of central islands due to masking occurring as a result of ablation effluent, later-generation broad-beam lasers have overcome these concerns with better algorithms and introduction of variable spot diameters.

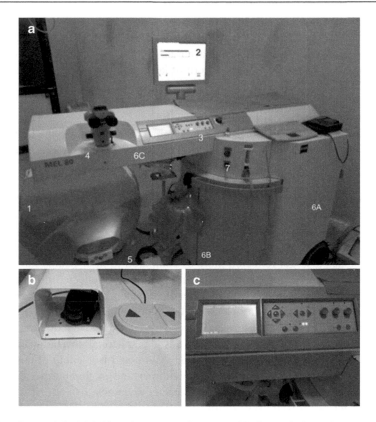

Fig. 13.1 Parts of the Mel 80 excimer laser (Carl Zeiss Meditec AG, Jena, Germany). (**a**) An overview of the whole machine; (**b**). Closeup view of the foot control pedal. (**c**) Closeup view of the control panel

Subheads in a:
1. Patient bed
2. Computer for data entry (e.g., refractive error, ablation depth) and planning
3. Control panel
4. Operating microscope head for lifting flap before ablation, irrigating the bed, and replacing the flap
5. Foot switch to control start and stop of excimer ablation
6. 6A Laser cavity: consisting of a laser head with high-voltage power supply, a trigger unit, and a laser interface

    6B Gas-handling system: contains a premix of laser gases and a flushing gas
7. Emergency stop switch (red button)

- **Variable spot diameter:** Circular beams of varying diameters are utilized, to perform the initial ablation with larger spot sizes **followed** by spots of smaller diameters.
- **Scanning slit:** Narrow slit beams of variable diameter are projected through a diaphragm to cause the ablation. Complex ablation profiles may be utilized by splitting the beams into smaller components.

- **Flying spot:** Small fixed diameter beams (0.5–2 mm) at high repetition rates (with the laser beam passing multiple times over the area to be ablated) are used. These systems need a sensitive and accurate eye tracking mechanism to maintain centration of the ablation. This pattern of laser ablation is used most frequently for LASIK.

13.2.1.2 Ablation Profiles

These may be categorized as conventional and advanced profiles, the latter including wavefront optimized (WFO), wavefront guided (WFG), and topography guided (TG).

- **Conventional ablation profiles:** In the conventional pattern of laser ablation, an equal amount of laser energy is distributed to the central and peripheral cornea, to correct the spherocylindrical refractive error (lower-order aberrations). Since the peripheral excimer beams fall tangential to the corneal surface, they become ovalized and also get reflected more as compared to laser beams falling on the central cornea which are perpendicular, circular, and reflected minimally. This results in peripheral points getting lesser effective energy (up to 80% energy loss may occur) with consequently lesser ablation of the peripheral corneal tissue and loss of natural corneal prolateness. This can lead to excessive induction of higher-order aberrations (HOAs) especially a positive spherical aberration which may lead to symptoms of glare, halos, double vision, and worsening of contrast sensitivity particularly under mesopic conditions and at night time. These side effects are seen especially with large diameter ablations.
- **Wavefront-optimized (WFO) ablation:** This ablation profile attempts to maintain a prolate corneal shape postoperatively, by taking into account the corneal curvature. A higher number of pulses and higher energy are delivered to the peripheral cornea to compensate for the loss in a laser energy seen in the periphery of the ablation zone with the conventional ablation beam profile. This helps to retain the asphericity of the cornea. WFO LASIK thus helps in reducing induction of a positive spherical aberration but does not specifically target the pre-existing HOAs in a patient's eye.
- **Wavefront-guided (WFG) LASIK:** Each eye has some optical imperfections (aberrations) such that a completely flat grid projected into the eye would be captured as wavy due to distortion of rays by the components of the optical system of the eye including the cornea, lens, and fovea. Specific combinations of these HOAs, i.e., spherical aberration, coma, trefoil, etc., can improve or worsen the visual function. Aberrometers can be used to detect these aberrations by mapping the wavefront of each eye. Most patients do not have substantial higher-order errors prior to their initial surgery and do well with aspheric ablation only. WFG LASIK also called "custom LASIK" was developed for patients with pre-existing significant HOAs (root mean square of HOA >0.3 μm) where information obtained from a wavefront-sensing aberrometer (which quantifies the aberrations) is transferred electronically to the treatment laser, to program the

ablation in a highly customized way. This is distinct from conventional excimer laser and WFO treatments, in which the subjective refraction is used to program the laser ablation. WFG LASIK thus utilizes a customized nonradially symmetric pattern of ablation based on the difference between the actual and desired wavefront in order to beneficially enhance each patient's "unique ocular fingerprint" and achieve a planar wavefront as far as possible. The disadvantage of customized treatments over conventional or WFO ablation however is that WFG LASIK ablates more tissue per diopter treated and also requires a more exhaustive and accurate preoperative work-up.

- **Topography-guided (TG) laser ablation:** This algorithm in addition to treating the spherocylindrical refractive error targets the corneal irregularities in an effort to reshape the cornea into an ideal curve. However unlike the WFG profile, the TG profile does not attempt to correct the aberrations arising from the crystalline lens or other ocular structures. Though initially used only for treating irregular corneas, this ablation profile is now also being used for treating virgin corneas with myopia or astigmatism.

13.2.1.3   Eye Alignment and Tracking

Flying spot excimer lasers and high-precision femtosecond laser systems necessitate the requirement of proper eye alignment systems to maintain centration while delivering the customized ablation profile. Such alignment is achieved using landmarks at the limbus as well as recognition of unique iris details (iris registration) by infrared cameras. Laser systems may have either passive trackers (where treatment is interrupted if the eye movement exceeds a certain limit) or active trackers (despite eye movement, using a sophisticated and complex mirror system, the excimer laser beam is directed onto the proper location on the cornea) or a combination of both. Table 13.1 enlists some common excimer laser platforms.

Table 13.1   Some excimer laser platforms

Laser platform	AMO Visx Star S4 IR (Abbott Medical Optics Inc., Santa Ana, California)	WaveLight EX500 (Alcon Laboratories Inc., Ft Worth, Texas)	Mel 80 (Carl Zeiss Meditec AG, Jena, Germany)
Type of ablation	Flying spot	Flying spot	Flying spot
Laser head repetition rate	Variable (between 6 Hz and 20 Hz)	500 Hz	250 Hz
Spot size	Variable size 0.65–6.5 mm	0.68 mm	0.7 ± 0.1 mm
Type of ablation	Conventional and Wavefront guided	Wavefront optimized, Wavefront guided Topography guided Custom Q	Wavefront optimized Wavefront guided Topography guided PRESBYOND Laser blended vision
Interfacing aberrometer	Hartmann-Shack	Tscherning	Hartmann-Shack

13.2.2 Photodisruption

The femtosecond laser is based on photodisruption and has applications in both LASIK and ReLEx/SMILE. This is a solid-state Nd:glass-focused laser that works in the infrared range with a wavelength of 1053 nm. Ultrafast pulses in the femtosecond range (100×10^{-15} s) are focused within the corneal stroma at a predetermined depth. Tissue effects are initiated by laser-induced optical breakdown (LIOB) where generation of microplasma bubbles of 1–5 µm size enables the target to absorb additional laser energy followed by secondary effects of shock wave emission and generation of cavitation bubbles. Contiguous photodisruption can help create flaps, channels, lenticules, and incisions in the cornea. Compared to lasers which work in the nanosecond range (e.g., Nd:YAG laser) and cause collateral damage because of the higher energy levels required (in the millijoule range), the decreased pulse duration in the femtosecond laser enables significantly lower energy levels and smaller spot sizes to reach the threshold for optical breakdown. This causes minimal damage to the surrounding tissue. Figures 13.2 and 13.3 show the important parts of two commonly used femtosecond lasers – the IntraLase iFS (Abbott Medical Optics Inc., Santa Ana, California) and the VisuMax SMILE femtosecond laser platform (Carl Zeiss Meditec AG, Jena, Germany). While the IntraLase is used for flap creation during LASIK, the VisuMax is a refractive platform for SMILE.

13.2.2.1 Patterns of Photodisruption

The pattern of laser pulse placement during LASIK corneal flap creation can be of two types:

- **"Raster Pattern"** wherein the direction of flap dissection depends on the location of the hinge, e.g., for a superior hinge, the dissection proceeds from the superior cornea toward the inferior cornea, the laser pulses being directed in a side-to-side manner from one end of the flap to the other. Conversely for a nasally situated hinge, the dissection proceeds from the nasal to temporal cornea, the laser pulses being fired successively from the superior edge of the flap to the inferior edge.
- **"Spiral Pattern"** where the resection starts at the center of the cornea and proceeds outward in the pattern of expanding concentric rings. Table 13.2 enlists some common femtosecond laser platforms. Table 13.3 compares the basic principles of excimer and femtosecond lasers for refractive surgery.

13.2.3 Photothermal

- Photothermal effects have a limited application in treating hyperopia and remain an evolving technology, not commonly used at present. Table 13.4 gives a comparison of methods of flap creation during LASIK-the microkeratome vs. the femtosecond laser.

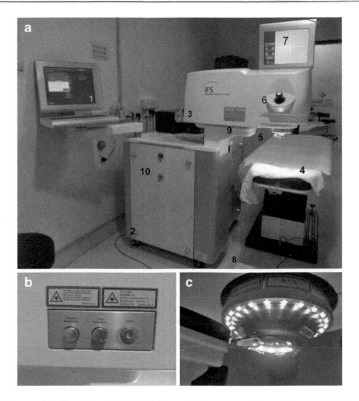

Fig. 13.2 Parts of the IntraLase iFS 150 Advanced Femtosecond Laser System. (Abbott Medical Optics Inc., Santa Ana, California)
(**a**: overview of the whole machine; **b**: closeup view of the control panel; **c**: closeup view of the loading deck with locking arm for patient interface)
Subheads in a:
1. **User monitor and keyboard:** laser resection parameters are entered, controlled, and monitored from the display panel and keyboard.
2. **Laser console** houses the laser assembly, electronic circuits, and cooling system.
3. **Beam delivery device** that focuses the scanned laser beam at a predetermined depth in the cornea with high precision.
4. **Patient table**
5. **Loading deck with locking arm** for patient interface: it is located at the output of the beam delivery device and couples the laser output to the patient interface applanation cone. The locking arm secures the applanation cone into position, preventing it from slipping out of place.
6. **Joystick** to control positioning and docking.
7. **Video microscope** with a high-resolution video camera to relay the magnified image of the surgical field to the screen. This view is required to utilize the user-defined treatment offset function, e.g., moving the flap in cases of decentered docking, as well as for a general view of the surgical field, while the treatment is in progress.
8. **Footswitch** (not shown in figure): actuation of the footswitch by placing a foot inside the housing and pressing down on the spring-loaded pedal is required to initiate laser treatment. Releasing the footswitch immediately stops the laser treatment.
9. **Control panel with three knobs:** one for **surgical illumination** (for LEDs mounted on the outside of the objective lens assembly to view the surgical field), the second for **cone illumination** (for the LEDs mounted on the interior of the objective lens assembly to view the applanation cone and the applanated cornea), and a third **home button** (to be used instead of the joystick to quickly move the beam delivery device from the surgical field following completion of a resection procedure).
10. **Emergency** *off* **button**

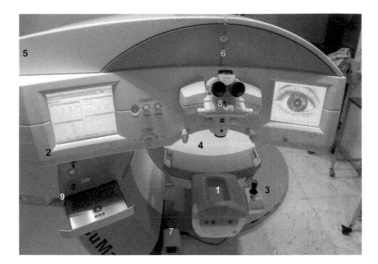

Fig. 13.3 VisuMax (Carl Zeiss Meditec AG, Jena, Germany): Components of the SMILE femto-second laser platform. 1. Patient bed. 2. Computer for data entry and visualization of procedure. 3. Joystick to control eye and PI placement. 4. Placement of suction ring of PI. 5. Laser housing unit. 6. Laser delivery arm. 7. Foot pedal to control laser firing. 8. Microscope for viewing, centration, dissecting the lenticule. 9. Emergency red stop switch

Table 13.2 Some femtosecond laser platforms

Laser platform	IntraLase iFS150 (Abbott Medical Optics Inc., Santa Ana, California)	VisuMax (Carl Zeiss Meditec AG, Jena, Germany)	WaveLight FS 200 (Alcon Laboratories Inc., Ft Worth, Texas)
Wavelength	1053 nm	1043 nm	1045 nm
Pattern of ablation	Raster	Spiral	Raster
Centration	Computer based	Mechanical	Computer based
Applanation surface	Planar	Curved, 3 sizes	Modified Planar
Spot size	1 um	1 um	3 um
Pulse frequency	150 kHz	500 kHz	200 kHz
Procedures	• LASIK flaps • Lamellar and full-thickness keratoplasty • Intracorneal ring segment pockets	• LASIK flaps • SMILE, ReLEx • Lamellar and full-thickness keratoplasty • Intracorneal ring segment pockets	• LASIK flaps • Lamellar and full-thickness keratoplasty • Intracorneal ring segment pockets

Table 13.3 Comparison of excimer and femtosecond platforms for refractive surgery

Laser type/properties	Excimer	Femtosecond
Principle	Photoablation	Photodisruption
Wavelength	193 nm argon fluoride (gas)	1053 nm (solid state)
Depth of penetration	Superficial only	Deeper, can be modulated
Incisions and flaps	No	Yes
Sensitivity to humidity, ambient air pressure, and temperature	Yes	No
Applications	PRK, LASIK, phototherapeutic keratectomy (PTK)	LASIK (flaps only), ReLEx and SMILE, Femtosecond laser-assisted cataract surgery (FLACS)
Platforms	**Star S4 IR** (Abbott Medical Optics Inc., Santa Ana, California) **WaveLight EX500** (Alcon Laboratories Inc., Ft Worth, Texas) **Mel 90 and Mel 80** (Carl Zeiss Meditec AG, Jena, Germany) **Amaris** (Schwind Esiris eye-tech solutions GmbH, Germany) **Nidek EC5000** (Nidek, Gamagori, Japan)	**IntraLase** (Abbott Medical Optics Inc., Santa Ana, California) **Femtec** (20/10 Perfect Vision, Heidelberg, Germany) **Femto LDV** (Ziemer Ophthalmic Systems AG, Port, Switzerland) **VisuMax** (Carl Zeiss Meditec AG, Jena, Germany) **WaveLight FS 200** (Alcon Laboratories Inc., Ft Worth, Texas)

Table 13.4 Comparing microkeratome and femtosecond LASIK flaps

Method of flap	Microkeratome	Femtosecond
Principle	Using an oscillating blade, a lamellar corneal flap is created, while the cornea is held under high pressure	Infrared laser pulses create adjacent areas of microcavitation at a specified corneal depth and define the flap – stroma interface plane
Flap shape	Meniscus	Planar
Flap/hinge diameter and Flap thickness	Keratometry, pachymetry, IOP, and blade quality dependent	Computer controlled
Thickness predictability	Moderate	High
Side cut	Shallow angled	Computer controlled, variable
Unique complications	Flap buttonhole, free caps	Opaque bubble layer, transient light-sensitivity syndrome, rainbow glare
Advantages	• Lower cost • Ability to create a flap even in patients with anterior stromal opacity/scar • Less induced inflammation	• Greater precision • Lesser risk of buttonholing, incomplete, irregular or free flap • Precise control of flap diameter, hinge width

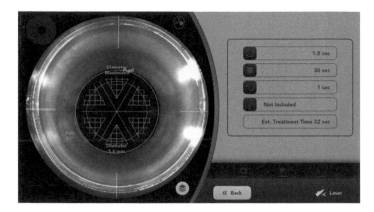

Fig. 13.4 The screen view of Catalys FLACS system (Johnson & Johnson Vision, Santa Ana, California, USA) showing capsulotomy (purple circle) and hexagonal nuclear fragmentation pattern (blue checkered wedges). Corneal incisions are not depicted in this image

13.3 Femtosecond Laser-Assisted Cataract Surgery (FLACS)

The femtosecond laser platform also has an application for cataract surgery for wound construction, capsulotomy, nuclear fragmentation, and astigmatism correction with limbal relaxing incisions or arcuate incisions. It offers greater higher precision and repeatability than manual techniques. These steps are performed in a closed-chamber, no-touch machine-driven technique and allow predictable results with less dependence on surgeon experience. Figure 13.4 depicts the screen view during planning of capsulotomy and nuclear fragmentation.

Suggested Reading

1. Stonecipher K, Parrish J, Stonecipher M. Comparing wavefront-optimized, wavefront-guided and topography-guided laser vision correction: clinical outcomes using an objective decision tree. Curr Opin Ophthalmol. 2018 Jul;29(4):277–85.

Basic Operating Room Machines

14

Mohit Dogra, Manpreet Singh, and Parul Ichhpujani

For achieving the complete surgical success, the surgeon needs to prioritize and address the problem of patients by formulating the correct diagnosis and treatment plan and performing a textbook procedure. This cannot be achieved without thoroughly knowing about your operating room equipments in an appropriate manner. This chapter briefly touches upon the "basics of common equipments" in an ophthalmic operation theater.

14.1 Ophthalmic Operating Microscope

14.1.1 Introduction and Principle

A microscope is a monocular or binocular instrument that allows visualization of structures that can't be seen with the naked eye. An operating microscope provides a stereoscopic, magnified, and illuminated image of the object to the surgeon via binocular optical eyepiece. It consists of two magnifying lenses—objective (close to the object) and eyepiece (close to the viewer)—that magnify the object under question. An illumination source reroutes light from the bulb to a point very near the

M. Dogra
Vitreo-Retina Services, Department of Ophthalmology, Advanced Eye Centre,
Post Graduate Institute of Medical Education and Research (PGIMER), Chandigarh, India

M. Singh
Oculoplastics Services, Department of Ophthalmology, Advanced Eye Centre,
Post Graduate Institute of Medical Education and Research (PGIMER), Chandigarh, India

P. Ichhpujani (✉)
Glaucoma Services, Department of Ophthalmology, Government Medical College
and Hospital, Chandigarh, India

© Springer Nature Singapore Pte Ltd. 2019
P. Ichhpujani, M. Singh (eds.), *Ophthalmic Instruments and Surgical Tools*,
Current Practices in Ophthalmology,
https://doi.org/10.1007/978-981-13-7673-3_14

viewing axis of the microscope and is projected down through the same objective lens used for viewing. This is called coaxial illumination and is an essential requirement in ophthalmic operating microscopes.

$$\text{Magnification} = \frac{\text{Focal length of eyepiece}}{\text{Focal length of objective}} \times \text{Magnification of eyepiece and magnification chamber}$$

The distance between the objective lens of microscope and the point of focus is called as "working distance" of the optical system. The objective lens and its focal length determine the working distance of a microscope. For posterior chamber ophthalmic surgery, the objective lens having the focal lengths of 150, 175, and 200 mm are used.

The field of view changes with the magnification according to the formula:

$$\text{Diameter of field} = 200 / \text{Total magnification}$$

14.1.1.1   Practical Pearl

The most comfortable position for any surgeon is achieved by allowing the target tissue to be both in the center of the field, at optimal point of focus with desired magnification. The neck posture of the operating surgeon is important to prevent long-term ergonomical complications—cervical spondylosis, neck sprains, etc. The microscope foot pedal is usually operated by the left foot (non-dominant), and a beginner should know it by heart.

14.1.2   Basic Components

The operating microscope consists of two main components:

• Optical component
• Suspension arm and floor stand

14.1.2.1   Optical Component

The basic stereomicroscope consists of a binocular head (Fig. 14.1), the objective lens, a magnification changer, and an illuminator which transmits light through the objective lens over the operating field. The binocular head contains two telescopes and adjustable eyepieces for correcting the refractive error of users.

Fiber-optic systems are preferred to transmit light as they produce minimal heat adjacent to the operating field and offer a larger field of illumination. The optical system may also include a beam splitter with a set of teaching binoculars to enable the assistant to simultaneously view the procedure. Some microscopes have accessories to capture the pictures and videos.

Fig. 14.1 Microscope head (*A*) assistant arm; (*B*) positioning handles with autoclavable covers (*C*); oculars with built-in scale to adjust the surgeon's refractive error; (*D*) scale to adjust the pupil distance of the oculars

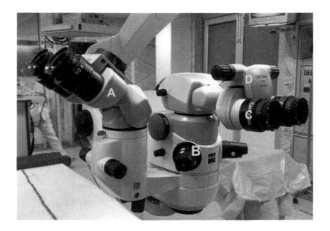

14.1.2.2   Suspension Arm and Floor Stand

The suspension arm holds the optical system, and the suspension arm is attached to the floor stand via a long column. With suspension arm one can position and fix the optics at intended place and level. The wheels of floor stand make it mobile and have the brakes to fix the microscope at one place. The surgeon controls the on/off, focus, position of the optics, zoom, and magnification with a foot pedal connected to the microscope via a wire. The horizontal and the vertical movement is also controlled with the foot pedal (Fig. 14.2).

14.1.3   Recent Advances in Ophthalmic Operating Microscopes

Ophthalmic surgical microscopes keep on evolving, and the latest advances are manufactured to integrate with existing equipments. Major upgrades include integration of the microscope into the surgical procedure and ergonomic designs. Some of the advancements are highlighted below. Modern operating microscopes are compatible with preoperative ophthalmic imaging devices. These systems provide image-guided overlays of patient-specific data and digital markers that can be viewed through the surgeon's eyepieces.

- *OPMI Lumera 700 microscope*: The OPMI Lumera 700 microscope (Carl Zeiss) allows 1080p full HD digital video on the integrated recording system. It also features a cordless foot control panel and an assistant microscope with separate magnification controls. For retinal surgeries, its proprietary noncontact wide-angle viewing system (WAVs), Resight 700 fundus viewing system, allows recognition of every detail of the retina. The Resight is equipped with an inner focusing system that allows the reduction lens set inside the microscope to be moved by the surgeons by using the foot control panel. This system holds two lenses, a 128 D lens for wide-angle viewing and a 60 D lens for magnifying images of the posterior pole.

Fig. 14.2 Foot pedal. (*A*)
Illumination intensity
adjustment tab; (*B*) X-Y
joystick; (*C*) focus tab; (*D*)
zoom tab; (*E*) light on-off

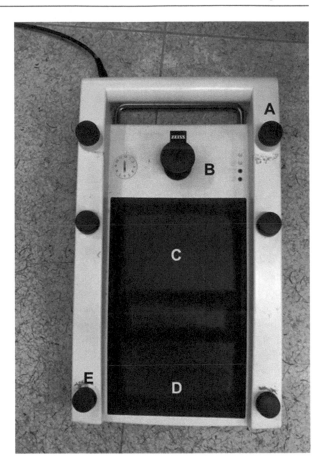

- *The Verion image-guided system (Alcon)*: This consists of a preoperative reference unit and planning device that capture and use a high-resolution image of the
  patient's eye to determine keratometry values, limbal diameter, pupillary size
  and location, and other biometric data.

  Surgical planning software helps surgeons develop treatment plans for the
  LenSx Laser System (Alcon) in terms of wound construction, laser corneal
  refractive arcuate incisions, toric IOL positioning, and IOL power selection.
  Some of these data can be fed into the compatible LenSx to program the capsulorhexis, wound, and arcuate laser treatments and to account for cyclotorsion
  errors while the eye is docked at the laser. After the laser treatment, the image
  and data are fed into the Verion digital marker unit in the operating room,
  where the device is linked to the surgical microscope. The guidance data can
  be displayed either on a 2D screen or through the microscope oculars of the
  LuxOR surgical microscope (Alcon). The Verion also includes wireless foot
  pedal communication with the Centurion Vision System (Alcon) during
  phacoemulsification.

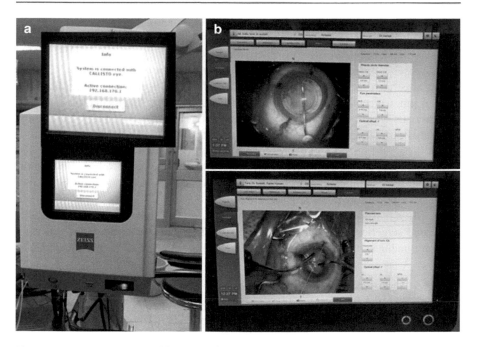

Fig. 14.3 Callisto system. (*A*) Microscope integrated with Callisto. (*B*) Screen showing markings for making capsulorhexis and aligning axis of a toric IOL

- *The Callisto eye (Carl Zeiss Meditec)*: The Callisto eye is a commercially available guidance system that integrates with the IOLMaster and the Lumera microscope. Callisto functions like a bridge: it links these two devices, thus allowing the surgeon to feed preoperative biometric data and plans in the operating room, where information can be displayed either through the oculars or on a screen attached to the microscope (Fig. 14.3). The surgical assistance functions include incisions/LRIs, capsulorhexis, and toric IOL alignment. The K Track feature is unique in that it lets surgeons visualize corneal curvature via a built-in keratoscope. This is useful in cases of corneal transplants. In addition, the system allows visualization of the biometric data captured preoperatively by the IOLMaster.
- *The Optiwave Refractive Analysis (ORA) system*: The ORA system (WaveTec Vision) device's image capture unit connects to the bottom of the surgical microscope and employs interferometry to measure the refractive state of the eye during surgery. ORA can capture refractive data about the eye in the aphakic and pseudophakic state, which are then displayed on a touch screen. The main advantage is that no preoperative biometric data is needed and keratometric and axial length measurements are done in real time intraoperatively. The data is shown as refraction with sphere, cylinder, and axis, and using proprietary biometric formulas and customized nomograms helps in selecting the proper IOL power for the patient. This technology is especially useful in long and short eyes as well as

postcorneal refractive surgery cases, where obtaining accurate keratometric values can be a challenge. Positioning of toric IOLs and placement of limbal relaxing incisions are also possible with this technology.

- *Microscope-integrated optical coherence tomography (MiOCT)*: MiOCT allows intraoperative acquisition of spectral domain OCT scans with a resolution of 5–6 μm. Currently three ophthalmic microscopes offer this technology, namely, EnFocus with the Leica surgical microscope, Haag-Streit MiOCT that is integrated through a microscope side port, and the RESCAN 700 (Zeiss), which is built on the Lumera 700 microscope platform (Fig. 14.4). In the RESCAN 700 system, real-time OCT images are projected on a heads-up display, allowing the surgeon to manipulate scan length, location, and angle through video monitor display or the foot pedal control.

MiOCT is used in retinal, glaucoma, and corneal surgeries. It has been used in retinal surgeries for conditions like epiretinal membranes, vitreoretinal interface abnormalities, macular holes, and tractional/rhegmatogenous retinal detachments.

Fig. 14.4 Microscope with integrated OCT

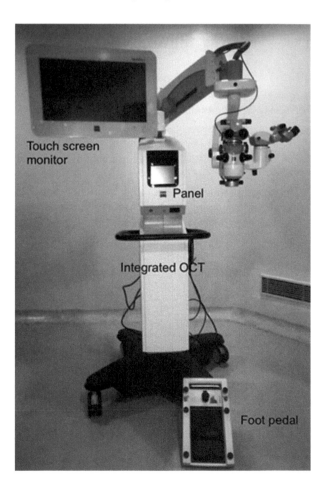

- *Four-dimensional (4D) MiOCT*: The four-dimensional (4D) MiOCT provides visual feedback through real-time volumetric imaging. 4D MiOCT allows for enhanced visualization of tissue deformation and instrument motion and decreases the need for constant tracking of the moving object. However, this technology is not commercially available at present.
- *Heads-up digitally assisted viewing systems (DAVS)*: These systems are stereoscopic high-definition visualization systems for cataract, glaucoma, and retinal procedures that display the surgical field of view in real time on a 3D flat-panel display in the operating room.

The NGENUITY DAVS (Alcon, Inc.) and TrueVision visualization systems allow surgeons to maintain a heads-up position instead of having to look down through the microscope oculars. NGENUITY hardware is comprised of a two-sensor, single 3D high-dynamic-range camera mounted in place of the microscope oculars. The cameras are connected to a central processing unit, which then projects the live feed onto a 55″ OLED medical display. The monitor is mounted on a stand, which can be adjusted and rotated. The surgeon wears polarized glasses to see the images in 3D. Reported advantages of this system include high magnification, improved ergonomics for the surgeon, a decrease in required endoillumination through enhanced digital signal processing, improved depth of field, ability to overlay MiOCT data, and enhanced teaching capabilities.

14.2   Phacoemulsification Machine

14.2.1 Basic components

Basic components of a phaco machine:

a. Machine, console, and foot pedal
b. Ultrasonic phaco handpiece
c. Irrigation fluidics
d. Aspiration pumps

a. Machine, Console, and Foot Pedal

The core of phaco machine is controlled by a computer with complex network of sensors monitoring the inflow and outflow of the fluids along with the delivery of electrical energy to the piezoelectric handpiece. The console is a touch screen monitor displaying the various parameters of phaco energy, aspiration flow rate, and vacuum settings with or without the bottle height (cm of H_2O).

The foot pedal is a vital component of the machine attached via a wire or wireless technology, to the machine. The amount of excursion or pressure over the foot pedal decides the action of the phaco tip - irrigation (step 1), irrigation + aspiration (step 2), and irrigation + aspiration + emulsification energy (step 3), in the increasing order. The side pillars of the foot pedal can be customized for the reflux or changing the steps of phaco procedure (trench, chop, irrigation and aspiration, etc.)

b. Ultrasonic Phaco Handpiece
- *Principle:* Piezoelectric property of specific crystals (quartz) which expand/contract to the electric current is used in the majority of phaco handpieces. Usually four crystal handpieces are commonly used as they maintain sufficient required stroke length even when any of the crystals becomes defective.
- *Frequency:* 40 kHz (27–60 kHz); cannot be altered for a specific machine
- *Stroke length:* 1.5–3.75 mill inches; can be altered by increasing the power up to one maximum amount (phaco tip excursion or the distance in the longitudinal direction at maximum power)

Practical Pearl
- The phaco foot pedal is generally placed on the right side of the table and that of a microscope on the left. The foot pedals are never placed beneath the microscope to prevent the surgeon's knee from inadvertently bumping into the surgical table during important foot maneuvers.
- In cases of a temporal approach phaco, one leg of the surgeon will be directly under the surgical table. Then the operating table must be raised to accommodate surgeon's leg, the operating chair should be kept at the same height, and the microscope should be raised for proper focusing.

c. Irrigation and Aspiration Systems

Irrigation is vital to maintain the fluid flow and intraocular pressure which help in removing the cataract lens particles and cools the handpiece (Fig. 14.5). Irrigation provides adequate anterior chamber depth which is commonly based on the gravity by hanging the bottle upside down from a fluid stand or a machine pole. Ideally, the fluid should flow into the anterior chamber at a proportional rate to the rate at which fluid is lost from the anterior chamber. The fluid is lost due to the aspiration and incisional fluid leaks.

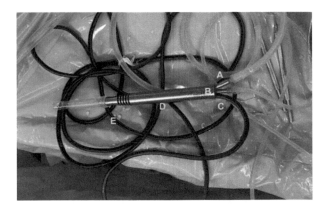

Fig. 14.5 Phaco handpiece: (*A*) irrigation port; (*B*) aspiration port; (*C*) cord; (*D*) stainless steel or titanium casing; (*E*) distal tip

Aspiration Flow Rate

- AFR is the rate of removal of the emulsified nuclear particles along with fluid and from the eye when the phaco tip is not occluded.
- AFR is measured as cc/min.
- AFR directly controls the followability of the nuclear fragments/pieces.

Vacuum is a force of suction created at the phaco tip by the pump, only when the phaco tip is occluded with a solid piece of lens matter. It helps to hold the pieces of nucleus close to the phaco tip helping in its emulsification. The negative pressure built inside the tubings sucks the emulsified material from the anterior chamber. Both (AFR and vacuum) are largely a function of the pump of the phacoemulsification system.

d. Aspiration Pumps

Mainly of two types: *peristaltic* pump (flow based, ml/min) and *venturi* pump (vacuum based, mmHg). The peristaltic pumps are designed as rotating rollers (4–5) which sequentially compress the elastic aspiration tubings. The rotation speed of the pump rollers is adjustable by the surgeon, and some pumps have an option to reverse the direction under command of the software. Thus, the surgeon adjusts the flow and the vacuum as desired at the specific step of the surgery.

The venturi pumps create a vacuum inside a rigid chamber as determined by the surgeon, and the flow occurs due to the fluid passing via the needle into the container. The absolute vacuum levels and its rate of buildup (rise time) can also be controlled. The modern venturi systems have built-in compressors.

Figure 14.6 shows a phacoemulsification machine with foot pedal.

14.2.2 Phacoemulssification Energy Mechanisms

- *Jackhammer energy:* It is created by the mechanical "to-fro strike" of the phaco tip against the cataractous lens.
- *Cavitation energy:* A low- and high-frequency cavitation energy is created by the vibration of the phaco tip causing the liberation of a significant amount of the emulsification energy. The implosion of the microbubbles near the phaco tip causes a release of 75,000 Lbs/inch^2 shock wave. The transient cavitation lasts only 2–4 µs and hence is short-lived, due to the rapid depletion of fluid.
- *Acoustic energy:* Liberated by the high-frequency vibrations of the phaco tip inside the anterior chamber.
- *Thermal energy:* Though less in amount, it is also postulated to play some role in the emulsification of the lens material.

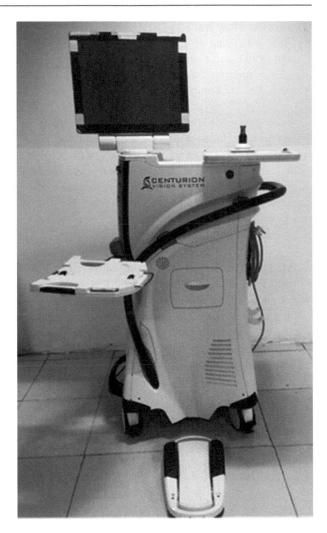

Fig. 14.6 Centurion phacoemulsification machine

14.2.3 Basic Phaco Power Settings

- *Continuous mode:* Delivery of the power is continuous with variations in power controlled by the amount of foot pedal depression.
- *Pulse mode:* The delivery of the power is in "on-off" cycles or pulse power delivery which increases linearly with the foot pedal depression. A greater will be liberated with each sequentially increasing pulse of energy. The time period between "on" and "off" pulse reduces heat and delivers lesser energy into the eye.
- *Burst mode:* Each burst has the same power, but the interval between each burst decreases as the foot pedal is depressed.
- *Hyper settings for power modulation:* Range of pulse rates (20–120 pulses/s) and burst width (4–30 ms) programmability has expanded for smooth and precise power delivery.

Practical Pearls

• Posterior capsular rent is more likely to occur toward the end of nucleus removal, where in the posterior capsule gets sucked in the phaco tip. Therefore the budding surgeons must always use the second instrument (a nucleus manipulator, *not a chopper*) under the phaco tip toward the end of the nucleus removal.

• The "epinucleus mode" with lower fluidics is suggested while removing the last quadrant of nucleus to avoid the vacuum-related issues.

Which Is Better: Venturi vs Peristaltic Machines?

• Venturi pump machines are faster; peristaltic machines provides more control.

• Irrigation and aspiration is faster with venturi.

• The followability is usually better with venturi pump but the latest peristaltic pumps provide similar effect; although venturi is better than peristaltic for irrigation and aspiration.

• The flow rate of venturi system depends on needle size (20G needle, 150 mmHg vacuum, and 55–60 cc/min flow rate).

• Peristaltic systems run at much lower flow rates (30–40 cc/min, 400–450 mmHg vacuum) with routine phaco needles. The chamber instability and post-occlusion surge can also be seen in these machines.

• When the phaco tip is occluded by lens material, the venturi and peristaltic pumps behave differently. To avoid the excessive built-up of vacuum beyond the maximum preset level, the peristaltic pump must shut off completely when the phaco tip gets fully occluded. Now, until the vacuum drops sufficiently below the maximum vacuum, the pump will not restart safely. The nuclear fragment starts to disengage from the phaco tip, as the surgeon breaks occlusion with ultrasonic energy, leading to no flow rate to hold the particle in place. In venturi pumps, the cassette vacuum is not affected by the breaking of occlusion with ultrasound energy. The fluid flow resumes when the phaco tip occlusion is broken in a venturi system. But surgeon should be cautious as venturi system can be aggressive (needs more experience). These days, phaco machines with dual pump technology are available (e.g., DORC associate).

14.3   Cryotherapy

14.3.1 Introduction and Principle

It is a technique that uses extreme cold produced by an instrument to freeze and destroy abnormal tissue. Application of cryo freezes the extracellular fluid forming ice crystals while the intracellular fluid gets supercooled (cools below the freezing point without forming crystals). Cell membranes are permeable to supercooled fluid, which flows out of the cells and causes dehydration and toxic buildup of intracellular solutes. This is followed by a thaw phase, which is equally essential for the destruction of cells. Intracellularly, a slow thaw allows for the longer exposure to toxic solutes and prolonged vascular stasis. Thus, a rapid freeze followed by slow thaw produces the maximum cell death.

14.3.2 Cryogens Used in Ophthalmology

- Freon—boiling point is -22.8 to -40.8 °C
- Boiling point of nitrous oxide is -88.5 °C
- Melting point of solid carbon dioxide -79 °C
- Liquid nitrogen—boiling point -196.5 °C

The carbon dioxide is the most commonly used cryogen because of its easy availability, but the liquid nitrogen is the most effective agent.

14.3.3 Basic Components

- Cryoconsole.
- Cryoprobe with insulated tubing (Fig. 14.7): various tip sizes and angulations are used for extraocular and intraocular indications.
- Electric supply to run the cryoconsole.
- Gas tank attached to the console through valves and tubing.

Fig. 14.7 Cryoconsole with cryoprobe

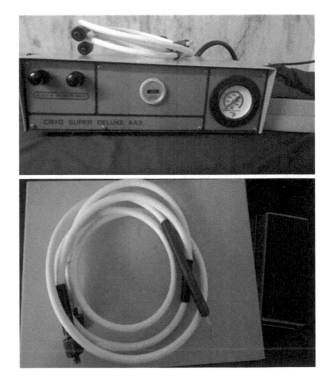

14.3.4 Indications

- Extraocular indications: trichiasis, eyelid basal cell carcinoma, ocular surface squamous cell neoplasia, recurrent pterygium, primary acquired melanosis of conjunctiva, and conjunctival melanoma
- Intraocular indications: cyclocryotherapy, cataract extraction during intracapsular cataract extraction, retinal break cryopexy, peripheral retinal ablation, retinoblastoma, retinal capillary angioma, and retinal vasoproliferative tumors

14.3.5 Complications

- Conjunctival chemosis
- Subconjunctival hemorrhage and conjunctival tears
- Corneal endothelial damage
- Panuveitis
- Retinal edema
- Subretinal exudation
- Iris atrophy
- Paralysis of extraocular muscles
- Sympathetic ophthalmia

14.3.6 Practical Pearls

- One must make sure that there is adequate gas in the cylinder and that connections have been correctly made and tightened.
- Before beginning, the functioning of cryotherapy equipment should be checked by depressing the foot switch and observing proper cooling of the tip.

14.4   Vitrectomy Machine Fluidics

14.4.1 Introduction

Pars plana vitrectomy has become the preferred modality to surgically manage vitreoretinal disorders, ever since Robert Machemer introduced it in 1971. Advancements in vitreous cutter technology, vitrectomy pumps, and duty cycle control have enabled microincision vitrectomy (MIVS) to become the standard of care in managing vitreoretinal pathologies. Figure 14.8 shows an advanced vitrectomy machine.

Fig. 14.8 Constellation
vitrectomy machine

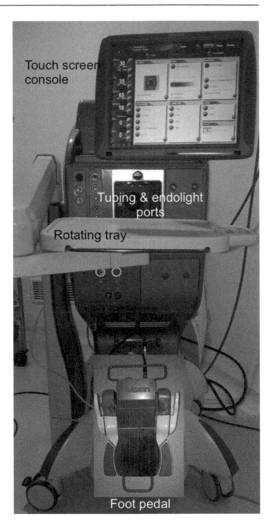

Table 14.1 Dimensions of various vitrectomy cutters

Gauge (G)	Diameter (mm)	Inner tube area (mm^2)	Port areas (mm^2)
20	0.9	0.350–0.352	0.254–0.306
23	0.6	0.169–0.196	0.122–0.173
25	0.5	0.128–0.129	0.066–0.125

14.4.2 Vitreous Cutter Technology

Vitreous cutters have evolved from electric to dual pneumatic cutters, which help in reducing the time required to perform vitrectomy. Decrease in diameter of cutters from 20G to 23G, 25G, and 27G have made MIVS the most popular mode of vitreous surgery across the globe (Table 14.1). Decreasing the size of cutters offers

Table 14.2 Common vitrectomy cutter settings with increased pedal pressure

	Cut rate	Vacuum
Proportional vacuum	Constant	Increased
Dual linear	Increased	Increased
3D vitrectomy	Reduced	Increased

advantages like shorter operation time, less postoperative inflammation and conjunctival scarring, fast postoperative recovery, potential self-sealing wounds, and less vitreoretinal traction. However, reducing the diameter of cutters does come with its sets of challenges. Of particular importance, as per Poiseuille's law, decreasing the inner lumen of the vitrectomy probe results in more resistance to flow and diminished flow rate. The decreased vitreous flow rate or so-called cutting efficiency observed with small gauge instruments is partially overcome by the development of higher cutting speed devices and high aspiration levels along with duty cycle improvements (Table 14.2).

14.4.3 Duty Cycle Control and Vitrectomy Fluidics

Duty cycle (DC) influences the fluidics during vitrectomy surgery. It is the percentage of open port time for each complete cut cycle. For example, 40% DC implies that the port is open for 40% of the whole cutting cycle.

Earlier versions of electric cutters had a fixed DC of 50%, thus maintaining a near constant flow rate. The original pneumatic driven cutters had a spring return mechanism wherein an air pulse pushed down the diaphragm within the vitrectomy probe, resulting in closed position of the port (the guillotine movement); at the same time, a spring was compressed that forced the diaphragm to the open port position. This spring return mechanism limited the control over the DC because as cut speed increased the DC decreased.

This was overcome in the modern dual pneumatic cutters, as instead of using a spring to return the guillotine to the original position, they use separate air lines foe opening and closing the vitrectomy port. This allows the DC to be controlled independently of the cut rate with customized modes.

Therefore, the surgeon can now have following modes in order to control the flow rate:

- "Biased open" or *Core mode*: Port remains open for the majority of time.
- *50/50 mode*: Port is open 50% of the time and closed for remaining 50% of the time.
- "Biased closed" or *Shave mode*: Port remains closed for the majority of time.

Newer cutter designs are capable of double cutting movements and are associated with a DC of approximately 100%. This leads to constant flow rates and shorter operation times, which in turn leads to less acceleration and traction on the retina.

However, irrespective of the gauge of cutters, as the cut rate increases, there is a trend to a 50% DC, regardless of the initial selected mode of vitrectomy.

14.4.4 Vitrectomy Pumps

- *Peristaltic:* Peristaltic pumps have inbuilt rollers compressing and dislocating the fluid within a tube, thus creating a gradient of pressure between the infusion and the point of pressure, leading to aspiration and directly controlling flow. Flow and maximum vacuum points are set on the machine prior to surgery. Once the occlusion occurs, vacuum starts to build up till the preset value, to maintain the desired flow.

  Drawbacks of peristaltic pumps include pulsatile vacuum, mild flow fluctuations, and inability to proportionally control the vacuum if there are bubbles in the tubing system.
- *Venturi:* Venturi pumps directly control vacuum to generate flow. The vacuum is created with air/gas flowing over an opening and reducing the pressure inside the ophthalmic cartridge. The flow varies according to the strength of the vacuum. A precise flow control is difficult to achieve, especially when changing the media (e.g., going from BSS to the vitreous).
- *Vacuflow valve timing intelligence technology:* DORC (Dutch Ophthalmic Research Centre [International] BV, the Netherlands) introduced the Vacuflow valve timing intelligence (VTi) technology that is capable of providing both flow and vacuum mode. It comprises of two small flow chambers (6 ml each), whose volumes are controlled by computer-based pistons, valves, and high-sensitivity pressure sensors located on the DORC machine, generating a fast vacuum response (vacuum set is achieved in 0.3 s) and flow control (0.1 ml accuracy), thus eliminating unwanted flow fluctuations.

The advantages of this system include the use of the flow mode while performing delicate peripheral vitrectomy close to the retina and vacuum mode for detaching the hyaloid.

Figure 14.8 show a modern vitrectomy system, and as can be seen in the image, most modern machines have a large touch screen graphical interface that allows for any easy transition from different surgical modes and a simplified machine setup.

The newer machines also have customizable, multifunction foot pedals. By using the foot pedal alone, the surgeon can change the settings and modes independently, thus reducing dependence on the surgical assistant. This new generation of foot pedals can be individualized for surgeons and can also be modified mid-case.

Nowadays, all the major vitrectomy systems are also equipped with full-featured anterior segment systems. Each system has the option to use either a phacoemulsification handpiece or fragmatome for lens removal.

14.5   Radiofrequency Cautery Unit

This machine is often used in ophthalmic plastic surgeries to provide a bloodless operative field or control the bleeding. It consists of a powered radiofrequency cautery unit (RCU) (Fig. 14.9a, b), two electrodes, and connecting wires. The active electrode (Fig. 14.9c, d) dispenses or "injects" concentrated current through a fine needle tip at a designated site, while the dispersive electrode "collects" (Fig. 14.10a)

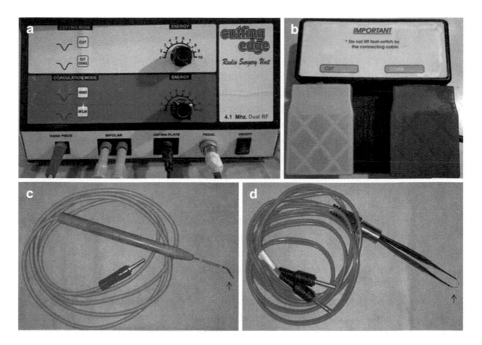

Fig. 14.9 (**a**) Radiofrequency cautery unit (4.1 MHz), cutting (yellow) and coagulation (blue) areas with knobs to control the amplitude. All the attachments are shown with power switch; (**b**) foot pedal with color-coded switches corresponding to the colors on RCU; (**c**) monopolar cautery handpiece (active electrode) with loaded empire tip; (**d**) bipolar cautery handpiece (active electrode)

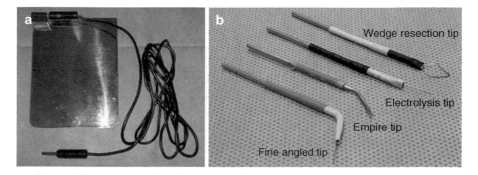

Fig. 14.10 (**a**) Body plate (dispersive electrode) to be placed in contact with the patient's body near the operating area; (**b**) variety of monopolar electrode tips

the same amount of current but from the larger surface area, hence no cut. Fine tip increases temperature, while the broad surface cools the electrode. Generally, 2–4.1 MHz frequency is required for ophthalmic plastic surgeries. The body of patient forms an essential part of the overall electrical circuit.

- *Principle:* Cellular radiofrequency absorption and tissue ablation
- *Frequency:* Unipolar (2.1 MHz, 3.8 MHz, 4.0 MHz), bipolar (1.7 MHz)
- *Radiofrequency generator (Power):* 90 W
- *Advantages:* More precise, less collateral damage, faster recovery, better hemostasis, safe

Based on Ohm's law ($I = V/R$), I current, V voltage, and R tissue resistance

The effects of electrical current over tissues can be *cutting, coagulation, and fulguration.* The waveforms of the current used for cutting is fully filtered, for coagulation is partially rectified, and for cutting with coagulation is fully rectified. In a cellular environment, the anions move toward positive and cations toward negative pole, converting the electrical energy to kinetic energy. This turbulent movement causes friction and liberates thermal energy. The tissue resistance depends on the type of tissue and its hydration—more hydrated the tissue, faster and stronger is the effect.

- *Cutting:* Low voltage and high current settings. A sharp tip or fine wire probe (Fig. 14.10b) is ideal; temperature rises between 400 and 600 °C for the very short duration. The cutting effect occurs due to the intracellular water evaporation and cell membrane rupture. The probe is kept slightly away from the tissue.
- *Coagulation:* High voltage and low current settings. Curved or straight bipolar probe is ideal. The heat denaturation of intra- and extracellular proteins cause the coagulation or desiccation effects used for hemostasis. Gripping the minimum amount of tissue and the small gap between limbs is advisable.
- *Fulguration:* Interrupted bursts of high voltage and low current. A small globular tip is ideal. Local destructive coagulation of tissue with charring accompanied by frying sounds is characteristic of this mode. The tip is placed slightly away from the target surface.

14.5.1 Indications

- To excise benign or malignant periocular skin lesions
- To perform an incisional biopsy from a vascularized mass or tumor
- Electrolysis of the trichiatic cyelashes
- To coagulate the arteries of extraocular muscles, orbital fat, etc. before cutting
- To excise senile or infectious conditions (xanthelasma, molluscum contagiosum, actinic keratosis, seborrheic keratosis, etc.)
- The cosmetic removal of a mole, wart, scar, hair removal, blepharoplasty, etc.

14.5.2 Precautions

- Unstable cardiac patients with a pacemaker.
- Eyeball protection while operating near globe, e.g., eyelid surgeries.
- Avoid using bipolar cautery inside orbit to prevent inadvertent optic nerve injury.
- Should not be performed very close to oxygen, can lead to an explosion.
- The patient should be in contact with the "ground plate" during the procedure to provide the best efficiency.

14.5.3 Side Effects

- Pain, tissue edema, and infection (coagulation effect on surrounding vessels).
- Relatively more scarring than with a scalpel incision, keloid formation.
- Hyper-/hypo- or depigmentation of the skin.
- The contaminated probe can transfer infection from one to another patient.

Suggested Readings

1. Charles S. Fluidics and cutter dynamics. Retin Physician. 2012;9:58–60.
2. Cushing H, Bovie W. Electrosurgery as an aid to the removal of intracranial tumors. Surg Gynecol Obstet. 1928;47:751–84.
3. Eckardt C, Paulo EB. Heads-up surgery for vitreoretinal procedures: an experimental and clinical study. Retina. 2016;36(1):137–47.
4. Goldberg SN, Gazelle GS, Halpern EF, Rittman WJ, Mueller PR, Rosenthal DI. Radiofrequency tissue ablation: importance of local temperature along the electrode tip exposure in determining lesion shape and size. Acad Radiol. 1996;3:212–8.
5. Oshima Y, Wakabayashi T, Sato T, et al. A 27-gauge instrument system for transconjunctival sutureless microincision vitrectomy surgery. Ophthalmology. 2010;117:93–102.
6. Rioux JE. Bipolar electrosurgery: a short history. J Minim Invasive Gynecol. 2007;14:538–41.
7. Spaeth GL. Ophthalmic surgery: principles and practice. 2nd ed. Philadelphia: Saunders; 1990. p. 41–55.